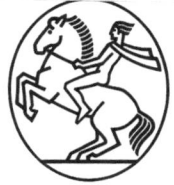

Stereotactic Neuro-Radio-Surgery

Proceedings of the International Symposium
on Stereotactic Neuro-Radio-Surgery,
Vienna 1992

Edited by
W. Koos, B. Richling

Acta Neurochirurgica
Supplement 63

Springer-Verlag Wien New York

Prof. Dr. Wolfgang Koos
Prof. Dr. Bernd Richling

Department of Neurosurgery, University of Vienna Medical School, Vienna, Austria

Typesetting: Thomson Press, New Delhi, India

Printed on acid-free and chlorine free bleached paper

With 101 partly coloured Figures

Library of Congress Cataloging-in-Publication Data

Stereotactic neuro-radio-surgery : proceedings of the international
    symposium in Vienna, Austria, October 11–14, 1992 / edited by W.
Koos and B. Richling.
        p.   cm. – (Acta neurochirurgica. Supplement ; 63)
    ISBN-13: 978-3-7091-9401-0   e-ISBN-13: 978-3-7091-9399-0
    DOI: 10.1007/978-3-7091-9399-0
    1. Radiosurgery–Congresses.   2. Stereoencephalotomy–Congresses.
I. Koos, Wolfgang Th.   II. Richling, B. (Bernd)   III. Series: Acta
neurochirurgica.   Supplementum ; 63.
RD594. 15.S735   1995
617.4'8059–dc20   95-3226
                                                            CIP

ISSN 0065-1419 (Acta Neurochirurgica/Suppl.)
ISBN-13: 978-3-7091-9401-0

Foreword

The past decade has been momentous for radiosurgery. After long years out in the cold, Leksell's brainchild was accepted by the neurosurgical establishment. It mushroomed in hundreds of neurosurgical centers; radiosurgical societies were founded; meetings, courses, symposiums were featured; thousands and thousands of patients have been treated; and a wealth of literature has been published. However, it is not at all obvious that the years since 1967, when the first Gamma Knife procedure was carried out, have been scientifically fertile. Nevertheless, it was a period of quantitative accumulation of data on clinical outcome – a kind of "product control" – that in due time will serve as a critical assessment of the place of radiosurgery in the management of cerebral lesions.

The present special issue of Acta Neurochirurgica edited by W. Koos and B. Richling includes reports presented at the International Symposium, in Vienna, October 11–14, 1992.

Being lenient or harsh in one's assessment makes the forword I was asked to write – a high risk venture. Nevertheless, the very failure to clearly define the essence of radiosurgery and the confusion today as to what its problems and promises are, provided the incentive to accept the invitation and give some thoughts and conjectures to this collection on radiosurgery.

As is usual in similar publications, the contributions are of shifting quality. Some of them present valuable material in an appropriate way. Others hardly achieve the level of scholarly treatment the topic deserves. Some authors succumb to the temptation to present material not yet matured.

What positively impressed me is the neurosurgical accent provided by a number of reports. They convey without explicitly articulating it, the idea that the Gamma Knife is no more and no less than a neurosurgical tool. The neurosurgeon should decide from case to case whether to use his microscope, or his Gamma Knife, or both. The two instruments are compatible and complementary. Additionally, they emphasize that surgical anatomy in general, microsurgical anatomy in particular, whether obtained by microscope or endoscope, are as important for radiosurgery as they are for microsurgery.

The volume includes also minor technical innovations as the use of intraoperative microspheres as indicator for subsequent radiosurgery and the immobilization of the ocular globe for radiosurgery in ocular tumors.

The present issue of Acta Neurochirurgica conveys the message that the trend in surgery is for procedures that induce minimal damage to normal tissue and preserve the function and quality of life. This aim can be achieved by technological achievements like Gamma Knife that transforms existing surgical practice, or it can also be achieved by improving surgical skills. Furthermore, it underscores the necessary interaction between microsurgery and Gamma Knife surgery, denouncing the shallowness of all gossip on the controversy "microsurgery–radiosurgery" that seems today to be an intellectual "growth industry". Hopefully, this heralds the future intellectual attitude in neurosurgery.

Charlottesville, VA, May 1995

Ladislau Steiner, MD, PhD
Alumni Professor of Neurological Surgery and Radiosurgery
Director, Lars Leksell Center for Gamma Knife Radiosurgery

Contents

Listed in Current Contents

Acta Neurochir (1995) [Suppl] 63: 1–4

Neuroanatomical Details Under Endoscopical View – Relevant for Radiosurgery?

C. Matula[1], M. Tschabitscher[2], K. Kitz[1], A. Reinprecht[1], and W. Th. Koos[1]

[1]Department of Neurosurgery, University of Vienna and [2]1st Department of Anatomy, University of Vienna, Wien, Austria

Summary

Both, neuroendoscopy and radiosurgery, are upcoming techniques in neurosurgery and become nowadays more and more important. In planning radiosurgical interventions it is very important to have both, the information about the morphology of the pathology itself, and also a clear understanding from the surrounding structures. Neuroendoscopic techniques gives the possibility to demonstrate well known structures without prior dissection. This paper focuses on these anatomical informations which might be relevant in planning further radiosurgical interventions especially in cases of the vascularization of the cranial nerves and the arachnoid membranes, these structures appears much more complex than described in "common" neuroanatomical textbooks. Endoscopic techniques also better demonstrate the real in vivo relationships and gives so a better understanding for interpreting "planning" MRI and CT scans. We therefore consider that neuroanatomical studies under a neuroendoscopical view are very important and could be very helpful in planning radiosurgical intervensitons.

Keywords: Neuroanatomy; neuroendoscopy; arachnoid membranes; cranial nerve vascularization.

Introduction

Improved visualization of intracranial anatomy with the introduction of the operating microscope a few decades ago has greatly diminished operative risks in difficult brain areas. A further step forward to minimalize the operative trauma is the development of neuro-endoscopic techniques. The use of these techniques in neurosurgery is nothing new. Since the beginning of our century endoscopes have been used during neurosurgical procedures mostly as diagnostic tools [4]. Currently these techniques have become widely utilized [1, 6, 8, 11, 12]. The development from the technical as well as from the neurosurgical point of view gives these endoscopical techniques interesting possibilities. The use of the endoscope in neurosurgery offers us many new options for minimal invasive neurosurgery. For the first time it is possible to demonstrate anatomical structures without prior dissection. Planning neuroradiosurgical interventions requires morphological understanding not only of the pathology itself but also from the surrounding structures. Endoscopic techniques better demonstrate in vivo relationships compared to open craniotomy.

Material and Methods

A series of 50 non fixed anatomical specimens were injected with blue and red LATEX via the jugular veins and the carotid arteries. Well known neurosurgical approaches were simulated including pterional, subfrontal and posterior fossa appraches. We used rigid and flexible as well as steerable flexible endoscopes with diameters ranging from 5 to 9 french and optical systems ranging from 0° to 110°. A xenon light source was utilized and the documentation of neuroanatomical structures and relationships was done by videotapes and colour slides.

Results and Conclusions

There are virtually no areas of the brain which have not been anatomically well described at surgical or post mortem examination [7, 10]. According to current trends in neurosurgery endoscopic techniques become more and more important [8]. Although using the endoscope also in neurosurgery is nothing new, only now these techniques are getting more and more accepted [4. 11]. In the literature there are some clinical reports about applications of different endoscopes. Most of them about applications in the ventricular system [3–5]. Only a few about using the endoscope in the basal cisterns [6, 12]. Treating intracerebral haematomas using an endoscope is also well described and discussed [1, 19]. So the terms "endoscopic neurosurgery" or "neuro-endoscopy" are well known in neurosurgery especially in connection with minimal invasive neurosurgery [1, 2, 8, 11]. In spite of all this it seems to be astonishing that reports about endoscopic neuroanatomy are very rare [12]. Especially in planning neuroradiosurgical interventions it is very important to have not only the morphological understanding from the pathology itself but also from the surrounding structures.

We think that endoscopic investigations of brain anatomy provide an in vivo look at anatomy while preserving anatomic relationships to a larger extent than open craniotomy (Figs. 1 and 2). Summarizing our experience from our neuroanatomical endoscopic studies we found that well-known neuroanatomical structures are seen completely different compared to open surgery (Figs. 1 and 2). Orienting under the endoscope is very difficult and requires both skill and practice. Structures rarely noticed in "routine" anatomical dissections become very evident. The arachnoid membranes and trabeculae appear more complex than previously described (Figs. 3 and 4). The vascularisation respectively microvascularisation sur-

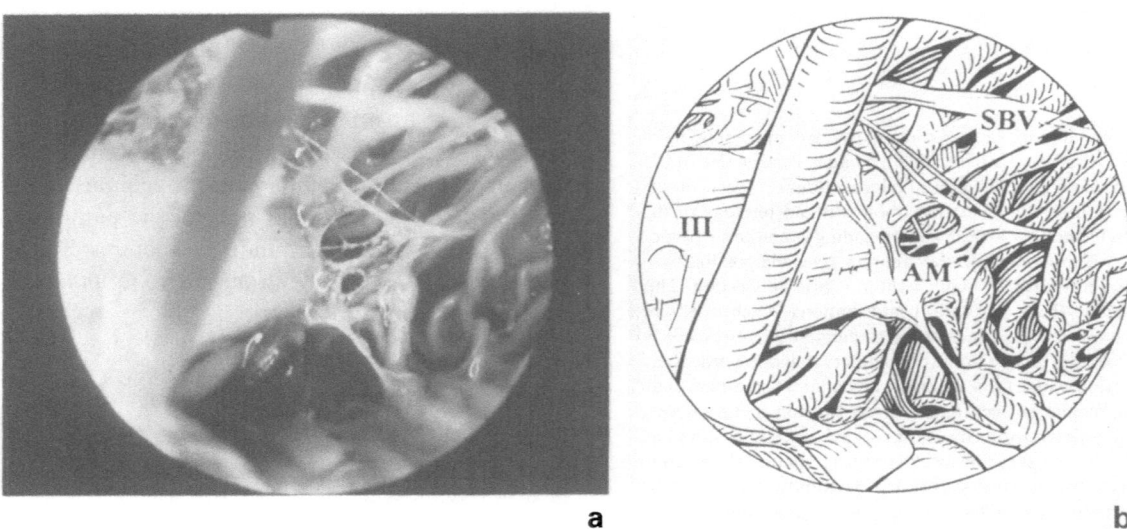

Fig. 1. (a, b) The origin of the right oculomotor nerve from the interpeduncular fossa seen with a rigid endoscope from a right pterional approach. *III* oculomotor nerve, *AM* arachnoid membrane, *SBV* short brain stem vessels

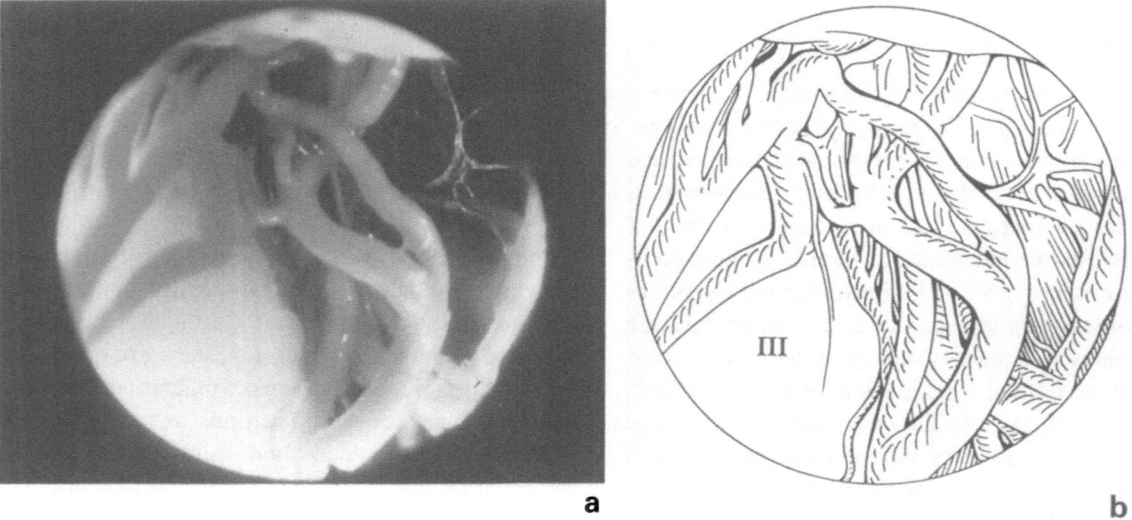

Fig. 2. (a, b) The same cranial nerve, but getting much closer with the endoscope. *III* oculomotor nerve, vascularisation of the nerve

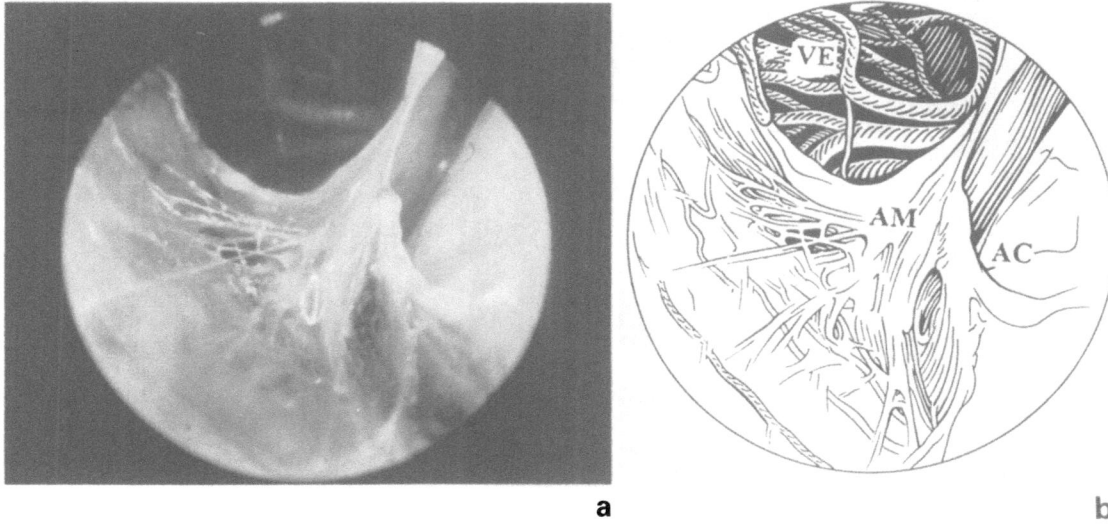

Fig. 3. (a, b) The arachnoid membrane and trabeculae seen from a right subfrontal approach by a rigid endoscope. *AM* arachnoid membrane, *AC* anterior clinoid, *VE* short vessels to the diencephalic brain

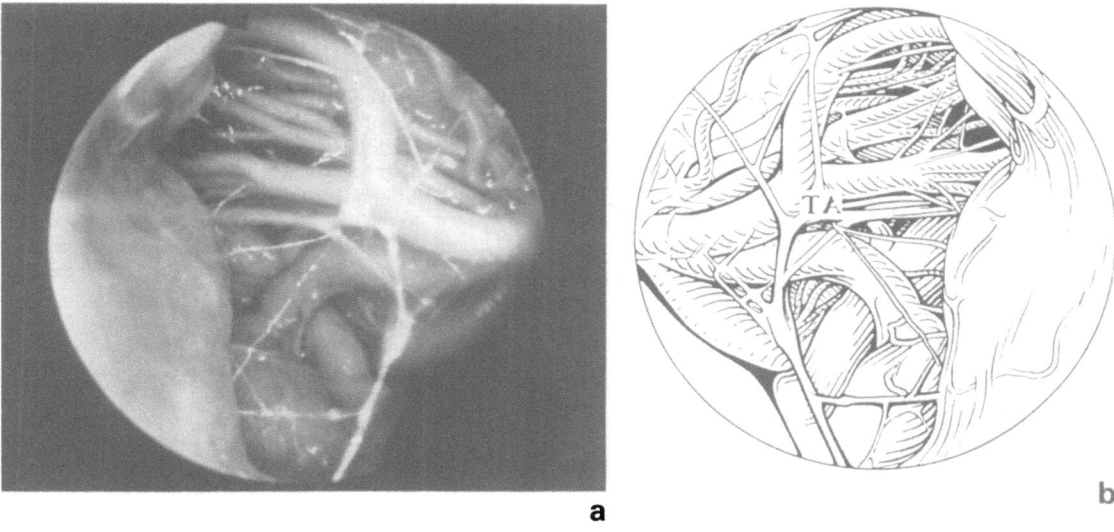

Fig. 4. (a, b) Arachnoid trabeculae and short vessels to the brain stem. *AT* arachnoid trabeculae

rounding the cranial nerves can be visualized perfectly (Fig. 4). Based on our studies this seems to be the limit between "normal anatomy" and "individual anatomy". In common it is well known from which greater vessel our group of vessels the vascularisation originates. But the "individual" topographical situation seems to be a kind of "twighlight zone" between a normal topographical situation and a real anatomical variation (Fig. 5). Individual anatomy especially in post surgical cases can be appreciated using endoscopy. The flexibility of the new generation of endoscopes allows one to "see around corners" providing information not available with current radiological technique while avoiding radical explorative surgery. The cases presented should demonstrate the usefulness of neuroendoscopy in demonstrating neuroanatomical relationships in difficult intracranial areas. The current diagnostic and therapeutic possibilities available with the neuro-endoscope are significant and exiting. Based on our experience we suppose that the endoscopical

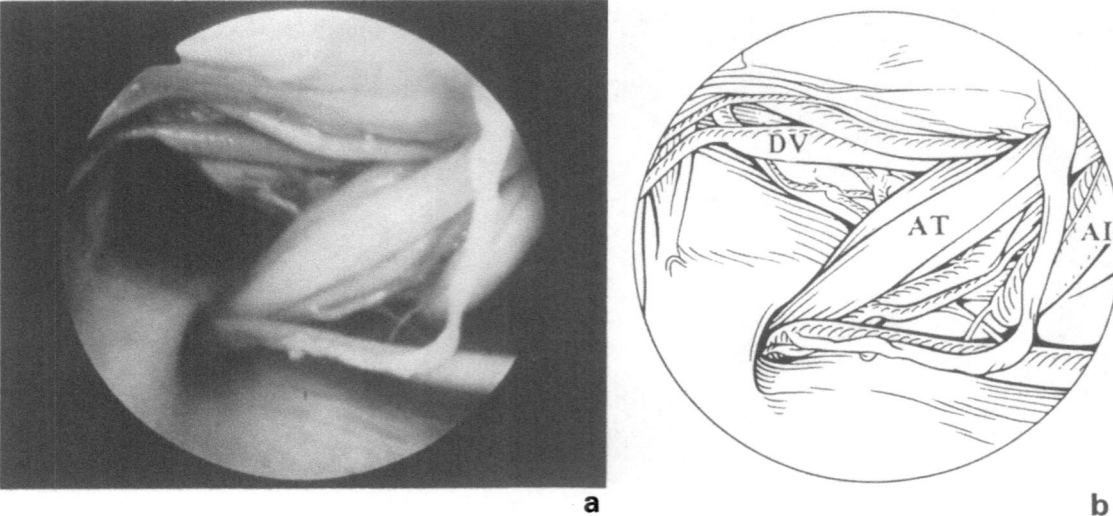

Fig. 5. (a, b) A view into the left cerebello-pontine angle from a left retromastoid approach through a rigid endoscope. *DV* Dandy's vein, *AT* anterior triad, *AI* Aica

view of neuroanatomical details might be relevant in planning neuroradiosurgical procedures. Beneath the well-known anatomical descriptions there is something like an "individual anatomy" and this seems to be the "missing link" between a normal topographical situation and a real anatomical variation as we have shown in the case of the arachnoid membranes and of course the real complex vascularisation of the cranial nerves. How much these details influence the outcome after neuroradiological procedures has to be shown in further clinical trials.

References

1. Auer LM, Holzer P, Ascher PW, Heppner F (1988) Endoscopic neurosurgery. Acta Neurochir (Wien) 90: 1–14
2. Bauer BL, Hellwig D (eds) (1994) Minimal invasive neurosurgery I. Acta Neurochir (Wien) [Suppl] 54
3. Caemaert J, Abdullah J (1993) Diagnostic and therapeutic stereotactic cerebral endoscopy. Acta Neurochir (Wien) 124: 11–30
4. Dandy WE (1922) Cerebral ventriculoscopy. John Hopkins Hosp Bull 33: 189
5. Drake JM (1993) Ventriculostomy for treatment of hydrocephalus. Neurosurg Clin North Am 4: 657–666
6. Fukushima T (1978) Endoscopy of Meckel's cave, cisterna magna, and cerebellopontine angle. J Neurosurg 48: 302–306
7. Gray H (1980) Gray's anatomy, 36th Ed. Churchill Livingstone, New York
8. Grifith HB (1986) Endoneurosurgery: endoscopic intracranial surgery. In: Simon L *et al* (eds) Advances and technical standards in neurosurgery, Vol 14. Springer, Wien, New York, pp 2–24
9. Kaufmann HH (1993) Treatment of deep spontaneous intracerebral hematomas. A review. Stroke 24 [Suppl 12] I101–106; Discussion I107–108
10. Lang J (1979) Praktische Anatomie, begr ündel von T.V. Lanz, W. Wachsmuth, Fortgef. v. J. Lang, W. Wachsmuth Teil 1, Bd1. Springer, Berlin Heidelberg New York
11. Manwaring KH, Crone KR (eds) Neuroendoscopy volume 1. Liebert, New York
12. Perneczky A, Tschabitscher M, Resch K (1993) Atlas of endoscopic anatomy for neurosurgery. Thieme, Stuttgart

Correspondence: C. Matula, M.D., Department of Neurosurgery, Währingergürtel 18–20, A-1090 Wien, Austria.

Acta Neurochir (1995) [Suppl] 63: 5–8

Intra-Operative Marking of Neuroanatomical Details – Helpful for Radiosurgery?

C. Matula, Th. Czech, K. Kitz, K. Roessler, and **W. Th. Koos**

Department of Neurosurgery, University of Vienna, Wien, Austria

Summary

This report is a list of simple but effective techniques for marking important structures intra-operatively. During the last 2 years in 52 patients intra-operative marking techniques have been used. In 37 cases a small piece of fat has been taken. In 10 patients it was done by a radiopaque Barium impregnated silicon sphere and in 5 patients with a piece of a monofilament suture. Postoperative checks were done by conventional X-ray, computer tomography and Magnetic Resonance Imaging. The indication in all cases was to offer landmarks helpful for planning postoperative radiosurgery. In case of fat and radiopaque Barium impregnated silicone spheres the markings were always well defined and clear in contrast. In those cases where a piece of monofilament suture was used it was impossible to get clear postoperative information. In general there were no intra- or postoperative complications. All markers were well tolerated and no side effects have been observed so far. The advantages and disadvantages of each of these possibilities are described and discussed.

Keywords: Intraoperative marking; silicon sphere; fat.

Introduction

Neuroradiosurgery is an important therapy to treat a variety of intracranial pathologies [8]. Often an open operation is not possible because of several reasons (the location of the pathology, the clinical situation of the patient, a radical resection of a tumor are impossible). In cases today radiosurgery is a well accepted method for treating patients safely and effectively [8]. There is another aspect especially in large brain tumours. With the possibility of postoperative radiosurgical treatment there is practically a new indication for operation, i.e. to decrease the tumour size to make postoperative radiosurgery possible. Further postoperative planning is often difficult because it is not easy to define the precise border between the tumour and surrounding structures. For the surgeon it is much easier to define these neuro-anatomical details under the microscope [3]. Therefore it seems helpful to make it possible to pinpoint important structures or to make out a topographical situation to make postoperative planning procedures easier.

Clinical Material, Methods and Results

During the last 2 years in 52 cases an intra-operative marking procedure was performed. Three different types of marking procedures were used. In 37 cases we preferred to take autologues fat. The fat was taken from the subcutaneous layer of the temporal region during the same approach. In 10 cases a small silicon sphere with a diameter from 1 to 1.5 mm was taken. The silicon spheres* are made radiopaque by Barium-impregnation (Fig. 1). In 5 patients a small piece of a monofilament suture was used. The decision which kind of marker was taken depended on the morphological intra-operative situation. The markers were fixed in general with fibrin glue and if necessary in addition with surgical. The documentation was done in each case by colour-slides or video tapes.

Case 1

This was a 25-year-old female patient with an invasive spreading pituitary adenoma. The adenoma was located in the supra-, endo and right parasellar region and infiltrated the cavernous sinus on the right side. The patient is without neurological symptoms with no palsies of the IIIrd, IVth or VIth cranial nerves. The only clinical signs were endocrinological with high prolactin levels. Because of medical problems it was not possible to treat with medication. The

---

* Barium-Impregnated Silicon Spheres, Art. No.: NL800-1005 (1 mm), NL800-1006 (1,5 mm). Manufactured by Baxter Healthcare Corp., 7280 North Caldwell, Niles, Illinois 66648.

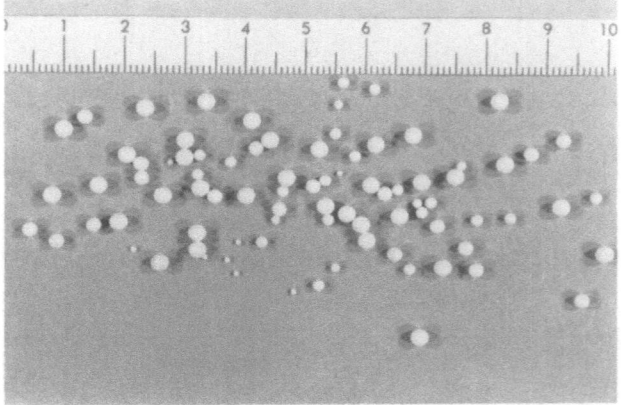

Fig. 1. Barium impregnated silicon spheres

tumour had been operated on twice before. The first time using a subfrontal approach the next time by a transsphenoidal approach. A radical resection was not possible and during the follow-up period a recurrence could be seen. We decided to treat the patient by radiosurgery. To make radiosurgery possible we decided to reduce the tumour by a subfrontal approach. During this operation the right oculomotor nerve has been marked with autologous fat (Fig. 2a). In the postoperative MRI scans the fat shows the position of the nerve (Fig. 2b).

Case II

This was a 47-years-old female patient with an invasive spreading meningioma of the left cavernous sinus. The tumour had been operated on twice before in another hospital. Radical resection was impossible. In follow-up series the residual tumour started to grow.

The tumour was too big for radiosurgery. So we decided to reduce the tumour by open microneurosurgery in the first instance prior to radiosurgery. A subtotal resection by a subtemporal approach from the left side was performed. A radical resection, because of the invasive growth, was again not possible. To make radiosurgery planning easier the left oculomotor nerve emerging from the cavernous sinus (Fig. 3a) and in the cavernous sinus (Fig. 3b) was marked using radiopaque Barium impregnated silicon spheres. Postoperative CT and MRI scans show the marker in place (Fig. 4a, b).

In general no intra- or postoperative complications were encountered. The markers were all well tolerated. No infections and no new neurological symptoms due to the marking procedure were elicited. Also no other side effects have been observed so far. In the cases in whom we used fat or the silicon spheres the marking is always well defined in the postoperative control- or radiosurgical planning CT or MRI scans. In cases we used a monofilament suture we could not get sufficiently satisfactory information postoperatively.

Discussion

Radiosurgery with the gamma knife is a procedure where narrow ionizing beams affect a predetermined target volume or induce a desired biological effect in the target volume without surgically opening the skull. This means a maximum of effect with a minimum of risk to the surrounding structures. For planning a radiosurgical procedure therefore it is very important to have exact information about the pathology and details about adjacent neuroanatomical structures [8]. According to this definition of radiosurgery it is clear that the more information we have during planning the more effective the treatment will be. Especially in invasive tumours such as invasive skull base meningiomas

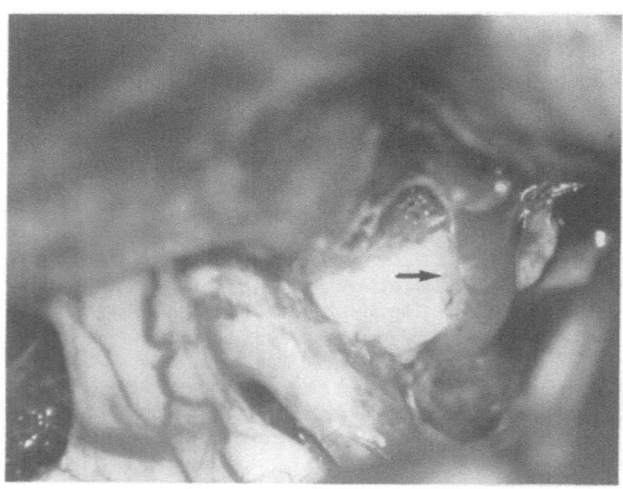

a

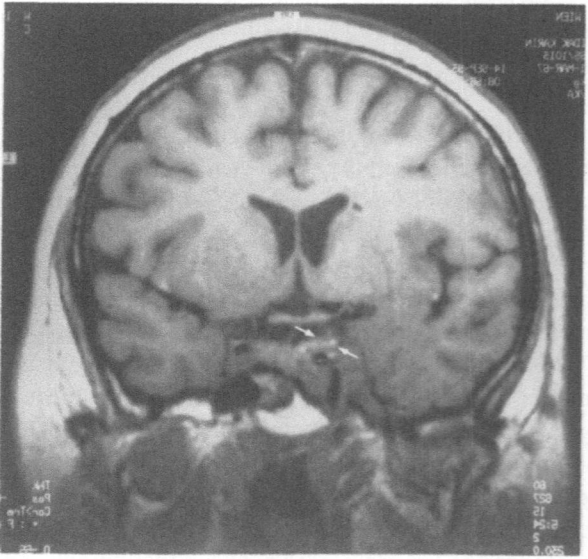

b

Fig. 2. (a) A piece of fat (arrow) under the optic (ocular) nerve. Intra-operative view using a subfrontal approach from the right side. (b) Planning MRI for radiosurgical procedure. Marked region using fat (arrow) and the oculomotor nerve (arrow)

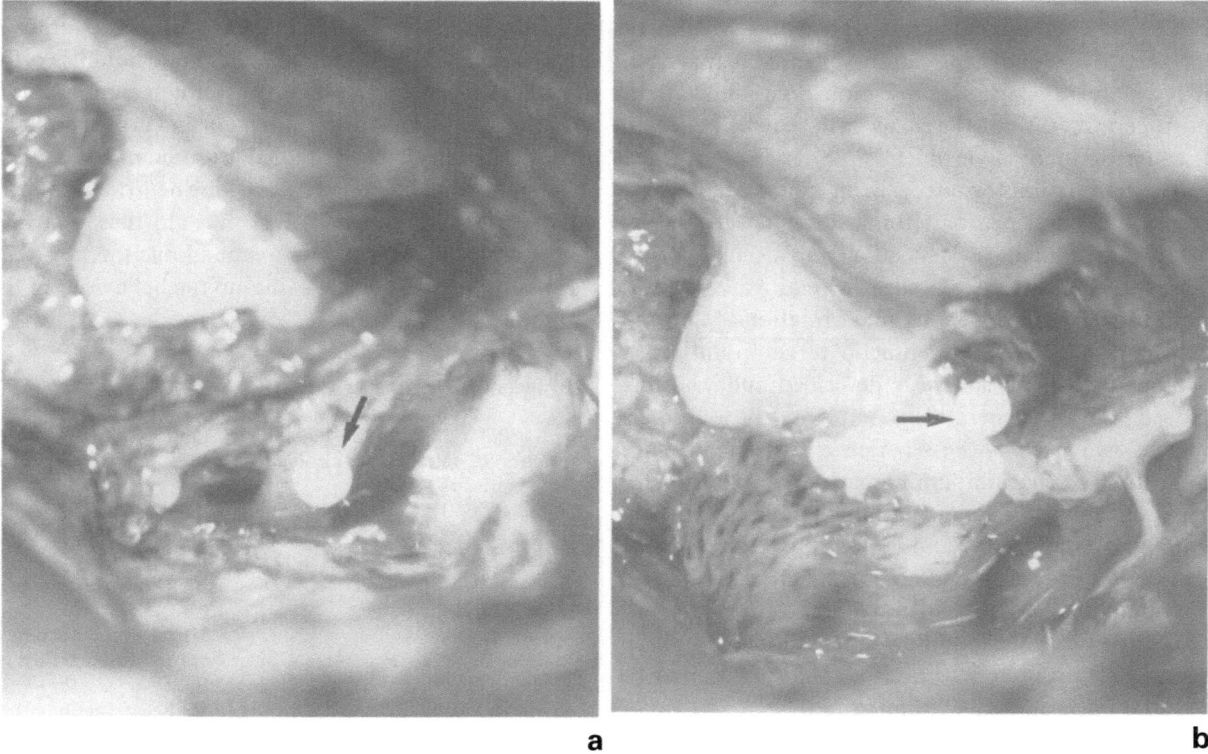

Fig. 3. Intra-operative view. A marker (arrow) on the left oculomotor nerve emerging from the cavernous sinus (a) and in the cavernous sinus (b)— the first marker covered with fibrin glue and surgicel (arrow)

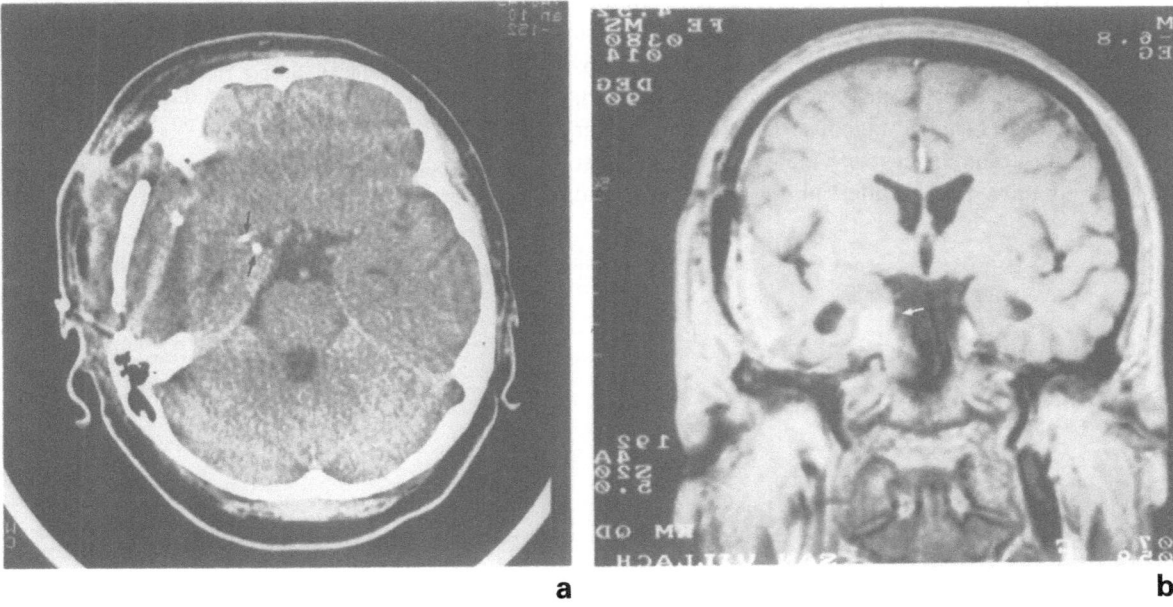

Fig. 4. Postoperative CT (a) and MRI (b) scans. Showing the position of the marker (arrow)

or gliomas where a radical resection is not possible [3]. Even when the surgeon thought he had removed all of the tumour it is widely acknowledged that many tumours are prone to recur [1, 5, 6]. In large, aggressive, locally invasive tumours we opt for "combined treatment" utilizing neurosurgery and neuroradiosurgery. The techniques we described in this paper for marking structures intra-operatively are simple but effective.

Fat is easy to manipulate around structures because of its plasticity. When using a transsphenoidal approach it is helpful to pack the resection hole with fat. In postoperative CT or MRI scans the fat can be well seen. It causes virtually no artifact.

The Barium impregnated silicon sphere can be used to mark a small neuroanatomical detail very nicely. They were originally designed for endovascular neurosurgery, where they were used for endovascular embolization of arteriovenous malformations [4]. Also the marking of the stereotactic target point by a radiopaque silicon sphere is described and well discussed [2,7]. In general these implants are well tolerated as evidenced by the experience with silicon shunt systems. The barium impregnation of the spheres makes them visible in conventional x-rays as well as in computer tomography and MRI. In MRI the spheres causes a signal loss and unlike metal markers (i.e. Titanium) they do not cause artifacts.

Using a piece of a monofilament suture has not been practicable. In none of the cases could the marker be found on postoperative examination.

It seems to be important to fix the marker appropriately. We therefore use fibrin glue in combination with surgicel. This secures the marker in the correct position. No intra-operative or postoperative complications were encountered. No infections and of course no marker dependent neurological deficit was observed regardless of which type of marker was used. Also it seems to be advantageous to document marker position by colour slides or video tapes. It is most helpful to have a clear idea about the anatomical situation and the position of the marker postoperatively. These marking techniques offer good landmarks for further diagnostic and therapeutic interventions. Information about the growing direction and growing rate of a tumour can also be obtained. In summary we believe that much can be gained by marking neuro-anatomical details intra-operatively. Not only do these markers enhance the postoperative gamma knife therapy, they can also be used for following-up the behaviour of the tumour in the future.

References

1. Adegbite AB, Khän MI, Paine KWE, Tan LK (1983) The recurrence of intracranial meningiomas after surgical treatment. J Neurosurg 58: 51–56
2. Alesch F, Hawliczek R, Richling B (1992) Marking of the stereotactic target point by a radiopaque silicon sphere. Technical note. Acta Neurochir (Wien) 115: 149–151
3. Koos WTh, Spetzler R (eds.) (1993) Color atlas of microneurosurgery. Thieme, Stuttgart
4. Luessenshop Aj, Spence WT (1960) Artificial embolisation of cerebral arteries. Report of use in a case of arteriovenous malformation. J Am Med Ass 172: 1153–1155
5. Marks SM, Whitwell HL, Lye RH (1986) Recurrence of meningiomas after operation. Surg Neurol 25: 436–440
6. Mirimanoff RO, Dosoretz DE, Linggood RM, Ojemann RG, Martuza RL (1985) Meningioma: analysis of recurrence and progression following neurosurgical resection. J Neurosurg 62: 18–24
7. Ostertag CB, Mennel HD, Kiessling M (1980) Stereotactic biopsy of brain tumors. Surg Neurol 14: 275–283
8. Steiner L, Lindquist C, Steiner M (1993) Radiosurgery. In: Symon L *et al* (eds) Advances and technical standards in neurosurgery, Vol 19. Springer, Wien, New York pp 19–102

Correspondence: C. Matula, M.D., Department of Neurosurgery, Währingergürtel 18–20, A-1090 Wien, Austria.

Acta Neurochir (1995) [Suppl] 63: 9–15

The Neuroradiologist's Contribution to Stereotactic Neuro-Radio-Surgery

E. Schindler

Division of Neuroradiology, Department of Diagnostic Radiology, University of Vienna Medical School, Wien, Austria

Summary

This publication is literally the same paper (having the same title and image material) which was previously presented at the International Symposium on Stereotactic Neuro-Radio-Surgery (Vienna, October 1992). Any actual updating of the topic has been avoided for reasons of historical accuracy and in order to document the atmosphere of that symposium which was then dominated by the unfolding of a new technology of intracranial lesion treatment. The neuroradiologist's contribution to this modality of treatment has to be the imaging and localizing such lesions accurately, as well as advising colleagues who plan radiosurgery and warning them about possible pitfalls. If there is no close cooperation between radiosurgeons and neuroradiologists, or if neuroradiological assistance is even disregarded, radiosurgical activities may fail.

Keywords: Gamma knife; imaging of intracranial lesions; neuroradiology for stereotaxis; team-work of radiosurgeons and neuroradiologists.

Ladies and gentlemen, first of all I want to express my thanks to the scientific organizers of this meeting for the invitation to present this paper. Entitling this I intentionally chose the word "neuroradiologist" – and not "neuroradiology". So, I am allowed to set forth my personal and quite subjective opinions about this topic. Leksell, in 1985, put forward this statement [5]: "In clinical practice brain imaging can now be divided in two parts: the diagnostic neuroradiology and the pre-operative stereotactic localisation procedure." Citing the creative spirit of this symposium I would like to emphasize that all I am going to say will be confined mainly to the diagnostic field and will not cover stereotactic procedures. I shall not go, neither, into particular problems of follow-up imaging after gamma knife therapy, since the pertinent experience here is very limited – the Viennese gamma knife has been inaugurated just a few weeks ago.

If an intracranial lesion is suspected, whether it could eventually be treated by radiosurgery or not, the neuroradiologist has the task of applying brain imaging modalities in order to answer the following questions as adequately as possible:

– is there a lesion (to be seen)?
– where is the lesion?
– can the lesion's margins be defined?
– how small (or large) is the lesion?
– are adjacent structures shifted or invaded?
– what kind of lesion is there (specific diagnosis)?
– is this lesion clinically relevant?
– are there further pathological findings?

It has to be stressed that this neuroradiological task must be based on clinical grounds, just as all our medical activities are. That means – the neuroradiologist must not cling to findings that are not relevant; on the other hand, the neuroradiosurgeon has to be aware of the clinical significance of the lesion he is going to target with his gamma knife. He must, however, try to treat the patient by shooting with his gamma rays at the lesion, and not anywhere else.

The neuro-imaging techniques for stereotactic procedures are CT, MRI, and angiography. CT seems to be the most frequently used modality at present, since there are still problems in MR stereotaxis that result from inhomogeneities of the magnetic field, nonlinearities, and eddy currents – so, always think of the risk of distortion when using MRI for stereotaxis. Poblems concerning the anatomical accuracy in stereotactic angiography will be mentioned below in an appropriate context. There is no doubt that the development of high-resolution neuro-imaging techniques has expanded the field of radiosurgery, since these techniques may precisely provide an anatomical definition of a tumour's margins. This conclusion, however, needs qualification – all the technical progress has not been helpful in this respect if there is an infiltrating tumour growth; in a lot of cases the tumour margins cannot be demonstrated since it has no margins.

Neuroradiology with stereotactic techniques is not only required for intracranial biopsy and endoscopy, but is implicated as well in many therapeutic procedures – stereotactic neurosurgery, functional neurosurgery (in epilepsy, pain, and movement disorders), interstitial and intracavitary brachytherapy, psychosurgery, and neuroradiosurgery. The important contribution of stereotactic neuroradiology to neurophysiological research should not be forgotten. With regard to neuroradiosurgery, reviewing the literature reveals that this therapy has been and is applied in many different lesions and also in mental diseases (psychoradiosurgery). These lesions are listed in Table 1 in alphabetical order intentionally not weighting the indication and value of the gamma knife for their treatment.

Since the pertinent and specific problems in different tumour types (meningiomas, gliomas, acoustic neuromas, pituitary adenomas, and craniopharyngiomas) and in vascular malformations will be presented and discussed by following speakers, I would like to demonstrate just a few examples of lesions in order to allude to questions that refer (at least in part) to neuroradiosurgery.

With good reason, MRI has superseded CT in elucidating the posterior fossa. Considering the diagnostic value of MRI in acousting neuromas, however, the

Table 1. *Application of Neuroradiosurgery for Treatment of Space Occupying Lesions*

Acoustic neuromas
Chondrosarcomas
Chordomas
Craniopharyngiomas
Gliomas (high-grade)
Melanomas (of the orbit)
Meningiomas
Metastases
Pineal region tumours
Pituitary adenomas
Squamous cell carcinomas
Vascular malformations

question is raised whether it is possible to discern and localize cranial nerves and vessels in the cerebellopontine angle harbouring a tumour – in my opinion, these structures can be visualized under normal conditions only (Fig. 1). So, impairment of nerves and vessels may be inevitable whenever the gamma knife is directed towards the cerebellopontine angle. Radiosurgery for acoustic neuromas with the hope of preventing hearing loss may be disappointing. I remember an interesting discussion in the literature [2] about the shifting of hearing loss from a retrocochlear to a more cochlear type after radiosurgery which was presumably due to an impairment of the internal auditory artery. Moreover, I think we are far away from definitely establishing the role of radiosurgery in tumours adjacent to cranial nerves, since the specific radiosurgical tolerance of these nerves as well as of the vessels is still not known. I do believe, therefore, that at present the

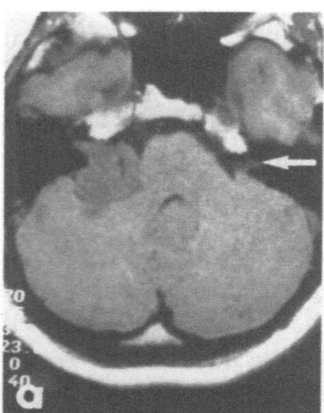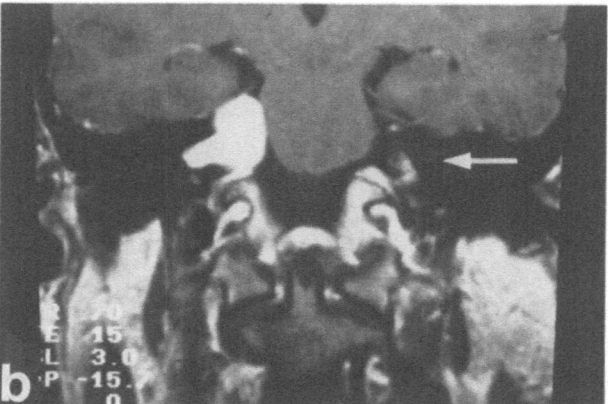

Fig. 1. MRI, T1-weighted. (a) Transverse, (b) coronal with Gd. Acoustic neuroma on the right. The normal nerve bundle is visible on the left (arrows)

gamma knife should be used to treat recurrent acoustic neuromas only and not be used as the initial treatment (primary tool) (except for very rare cases).

Figure 2 shows a parasellar meningioma which has encased the carotid artery and involved the cavernous sinus. The distance between the tumour and the chiasma is of decisive importance if one envisages radiosurgery in suprasellar tumours [12]. In this particular case (Fig. 2) the tumour is distant enough from the chiasma and treatment might therefore be possible. What about, however, the small vessels that supply the chiasma? Regarding the biological effect of the gamma rays, there are two mechanisms assumed – irreparable cell damage and/or delayed vascular obliteration. If obliteration of the small chiasmal vessels occurs, visual disturbances will result. Another question is that concerning the destiny of the oculomotor function in parasellar tumours – this, however, applies to the problems of both radiosurgery and microsurgery in this region.

In Fig. 3 a pineal region tumour is visible which turned out to be a germinoma. There is no doubt that a germinoma will completely disappear after application of the gamma knife. There is, however, a suprasellar tumour seeding (a rather frequent feature of germinomas) which must not be overlooked when radiosurgery is planned.

A complete and accurate neuroradiological examination is prerequisite when intracranial metastases are suspected and gamma knife treatment is considered. The computertomograms copied in Fig. 4 were made some days after gamma knife treatment of a bronchial carcinoma metastasis in the temporal lobe (Fig. 4a). A second and presumable third metastasis (Fig. 4b)

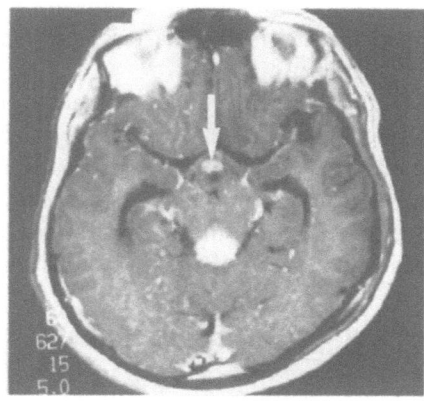

Fig. 3. MRI, T1-weighted; transverse with Gd. Germinoma in the pineal region with suprasellar tumour seeding (arrow)

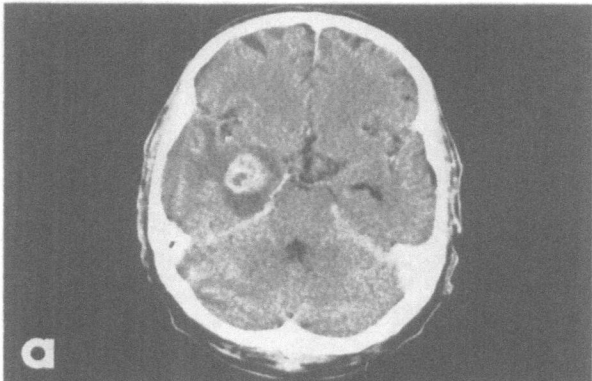

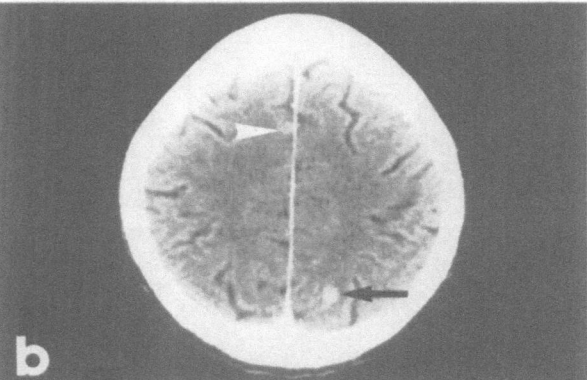

Fig. 4. CT, (a) and (b) after intravenous contrast. Bronchial carcinoma metastasis in the right temporal lobe. Further metastases in the left parieto-occipital (arrow) and probably in the right frontoparietal (arrowhead) region

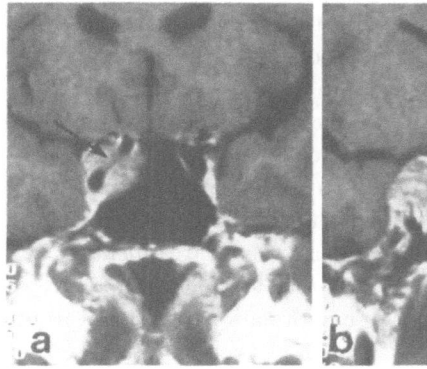 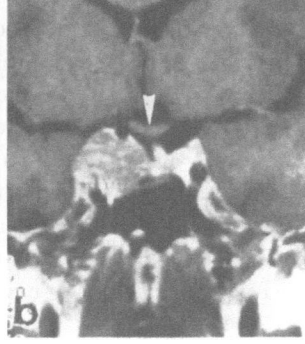

Fig. 2. MRI, T1-weighted. (a, b) Coronal with Gd. Meningioma involving the right cavernous sinus. The right internal carotid artery (arrow) is encased, the chiasma (arrowhead) is distant from the tumour

were apparently not taken into account when radiosurgery was planned in this case. In another case from our material, CT revealed bleeding of a rather large metastasis after gamma knife application – so, we must keep in mind that small metastases only are suitable for radiosurgery.

What about the role of the gamma knife in malignant gliomas? I am sure that there will be a certain use for radiosurgery following neurosurgery in tumours like the rather well demarcated glioblastoma shown in Fig. 5a. After tumour excision gamma knife treatment was planned (Fig. 5b). Four months after this therapy,

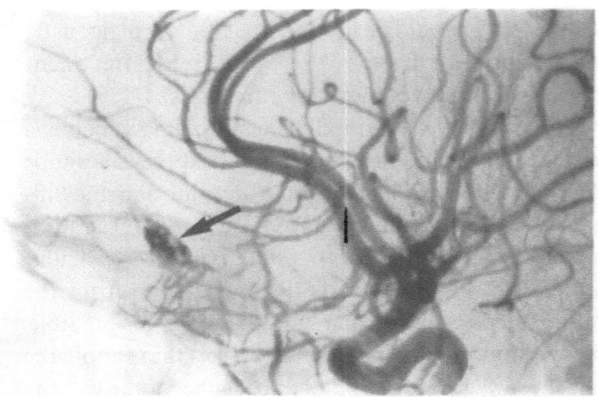

Fig. 6. Left carotid angiogram (subtraction). Small frontal vascular malformation (arrow)

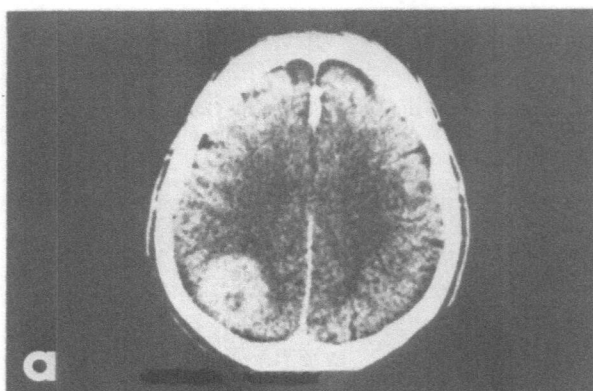

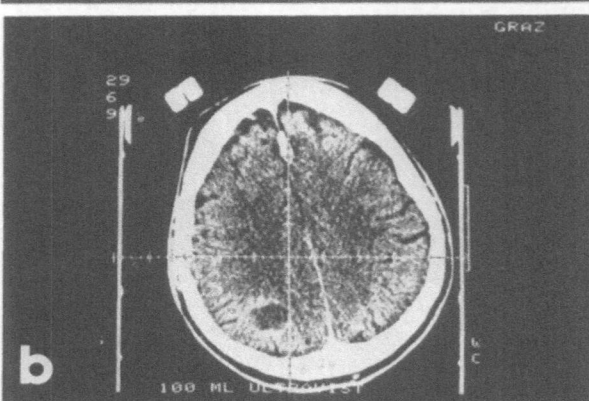

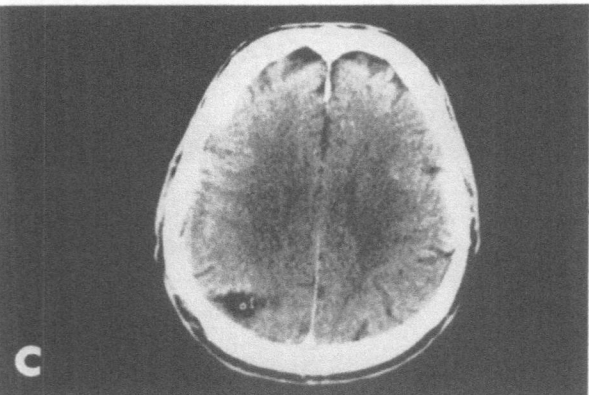

Fig. 5. CT, (a–c) after intravenous contrast. Parieto-occipital glioblastoma on the right. (a) Pre-operative CT; (b) stereotactive postoperative CT for radiosurgical planning; (c) follow-up CT four months after gamma knife treatment

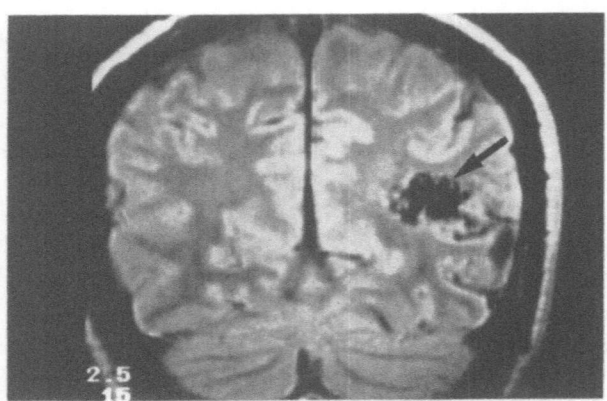

Fig. 7. MRI, proton density weighted; coronal. Vascular malformation (arrow)

there were no signs of tumour growth (Fig. 5c). For the image material of this case I am indebted to Dr. Pendl from Graz; in this context it has to be mentioned that the first gamma knife in our country has been established in Graz six months ago – Dr. Pendl, therefore, has a half-year radiosurgical experience.

The angiogram of a vascular malformation shown in Fig. 6 is very old – it nearly dates from the year when the honorary president of this meeting, Dr. Steiner, was the first to use the gamma knife for treatment of such a lesion which was in March 1970 [11]. With MRI, of course, small vascular malformations can also be delineated (Fig. 7). Which method, then, is to be used for diagnosing intracranial arteriovenous malformations which are possibly eligible for radiosurgery? Apart from the patient's clinical condition and his age, the following criteria determine the selection for radiosurgical treatment of an arteriovenous malformation (AVM): size and site of the AVM, feeding arteries, and draining veins. With reference to these criteria, angiography is obviously necessary for the assessment of AVMs. It is evident, as well, that stereotactic angiography has to be used for radiosurgical planning [9]. There are, however, limitations due to principles of ray geometry and projection which are pointed out conclusively in a recent paper of a study group from Florida [10]. Moreover, it is difficult – for the beginner at least – to achieve correct projections of the stereotactic frame. We fortunately overcame this problem within a rather short learning time, as demonstrated with one of our early stereotactic angiograms (Fig. 8). Neuroradiological contribution is also required for evaluating the result after stereotactic radiosurgery of AVMs [1, 3]. The timing of the neuroradiological follow-up, however, is debatable, as well as the adequate imaging modality. It seems advisable – provided the patient's clinical course does not require another strategy – to carry out MRI studies at six month-intervals, and angiography two years after radiotherapy [8] which should be the final examination if there is definite treatment success. Angiographic criteria for successful radiosurgery are normal circulation time, complete absence of pathological vessels in the former nidus, and disappearance or normalization of draining veins [6].

A vascular malformation which cannot be visualized by angiography is a challenge concerning both the neurosurgeon and the radiosurgeon. According to Lobato *et al.* [7] who collected histologically verified cases from the literature and from their own material,

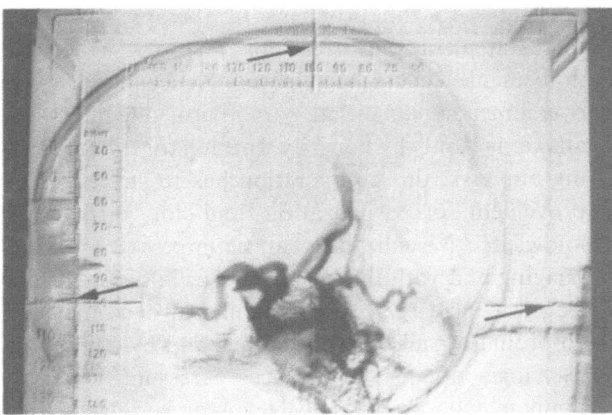

Fig. 8. Left vertebral stereotactic angiogram for radiosurgical planning of a vascular malformation in the posterior fossa. The stereotactic frame is correctly projected (arrows)

the so-called "angiographically occult intracranial vascular malformations" comprise arteriovenous malformations (44%), cavernous angiomas (31%), venous angiomas (10%), capillary telangiectases (4%), and mixed or unclassified angiomas (11%). I will not go into the hard therapeutic problems that are due to the fact that many of these angiographically occult angiomas are situated in or near the brainstem [4], I just would like to demonstrate the brain images (Fig. 9) of a 24-year-old woman; cavernous angiomas were histologically verified in this case – contrary to MRI (Fig. 9d), two cavernous angiomas are not visualized with CT (Fig. 9b). This case may lead over to the problem of choosing the adequate imaging modality which applies as well to diagnostic as to stereotactic procedures.

For any stereotactic procedure, this choice must be based on the following demands on an imaging system:

– visualization with accurate resolution (contrast and space),
– stereometric precision,
– instruments to adequately depict reference marks,
– reliable calculation programs,
– suitability for the patient.

One should constantly be aware, however, of sources of error when imaging the brain for stereotactic purposes – such errors may be due to intrinsic physical principles (e.g. inhomogeneities of the magnetic field in MRI), to equipment deficiency or fault (a defective feeding mechanism of the CT couch may result in a considerable mistake), to inadequate algorithm, or due to human failures. Human failures should never be disregarded, and prejudice and emotion can be most dangerous. So, if someone believes he can discern the margins of an infiltrating tumour since he wants the patient to be treated with the gamma knife since a gamma knife is available, the whole action goes wrong. In this context, let me say my very modest opinion that publicly claiming a third gamma knife for our small country is a rather dubious statement. Be that as it may – the most momentous errors are those whose possible occurrence we do not consider.

Let me summarize now the neuroradiologist's contribution to neuroradiosurgery. His task is the visualization of the brain using the optimal imaging modality in order to prove or exclude a lesion. He has, as well, to demonstrate the lesion's size and site and its margins, and to provide information about the adjacent structures and about further pathological findings if present. In stereotactic imaging the neuroradiologist's contribution comprises the choice of the appropriate method

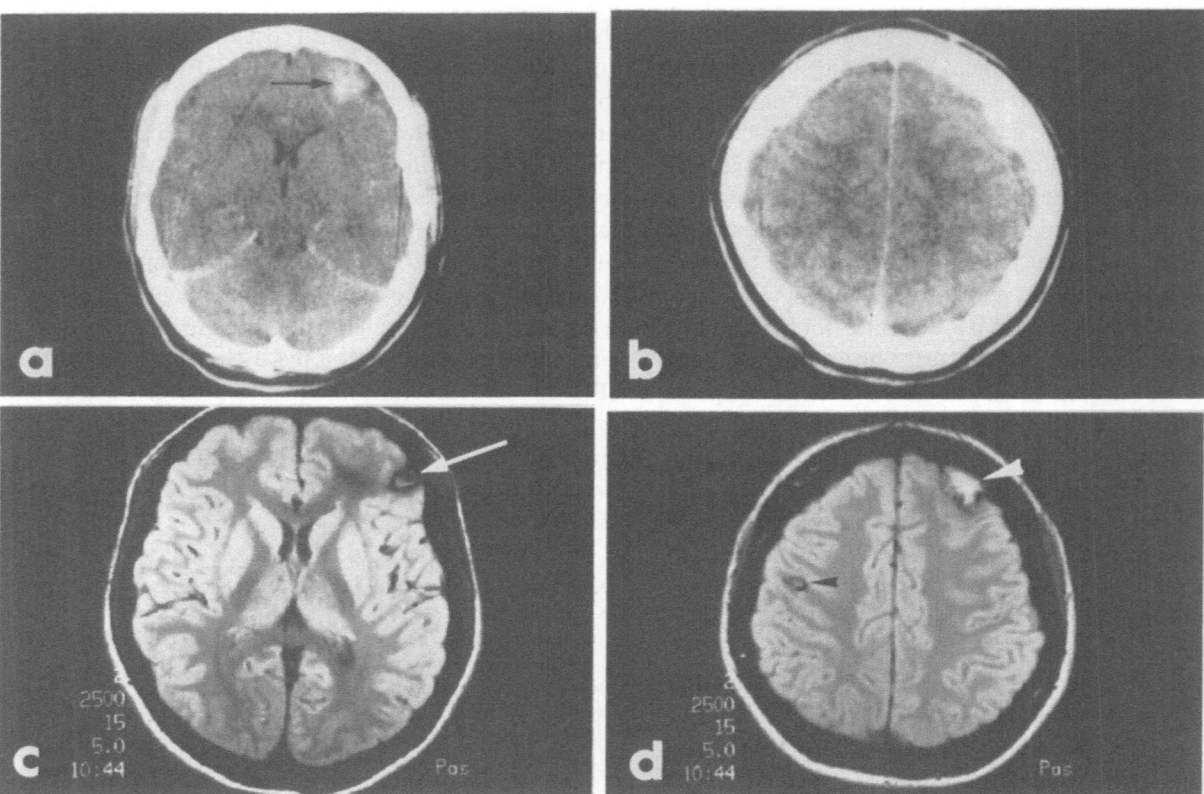

Fig. 9. (a, b) CT, after intravenous contrast, (c, d) MRI, proton density weighted. Cavernous angiomas. The left frontal angioma (arrows) is visible on CT as well as on MRI, whereas the left frontoparietal and the right parietal angiomas (arrowheads) are visualized with MRI only

and the assessment of the stereotactic precision as well. For follow-up after radiosurgery he should advise the timing of the control studies, and he has to carry out such controls with optimal imaging in order to exclude or prove remnants or recurrence. Referring to the neuroradiologist's co-operative function, however, the scope of his contribution is – or should be, at least – more extensive. It is my strong opinion that the neuroradiologist has to be involved in the discussion of the clinical relevance of the findings and has to contribute to prognostic considerations as well. His arguments concerning a lesion's nature should not be disregarded, nor his suggestion of further examinations that may be decisive. The neuroradiologist has to be consulted when radiosurgical therapy is discussed, and his warning against pitfalls should be appreciated. No constructive discussion, however, can take place if a neurosurgeon thinks himself to be capable of commanding the whole field and pronounces with arbitrary presumption the sentence: "This patient is for gamma knife."

May I conclude my personal contribution to the whole topic with comments on two statements. Firstly

– one can only perceive something which one knows; secondly – one cannot know anything that is not visualized. The first statement is one axiom of one theory of cognition, it concerns mainly the possible experience in our optical world and may be applicable to our diagnostic considerations, whereas the second one is applicable to the problems of therapy. Now, if these statements were irrefutable, no progress – neither in medicine – could be achieved. Hence, how can we overcome the somewhat paradoxical dilemma? The answer is – only by honestly working together. Focusing our task, this co-operation has to strive for improvement of visualization and for increase of knowledge. Visualization can be improved by skilful imaging and with the progress of technology. Knowledge will increase by co-operation of all of us in loyalty, co-ordinating all our endeavours, and by continuous exchange of our experience. Stressing loyalty I thank my neuroradiological team for its diligent assistance, and stressing experience exchange I am sure that this symposium will successfully yield considerable results.

References

1. Dawson RC 3rd, Tarr R W, Hecht ST, Jungreis CA, Lunsford LD, Coffey RJ, Horton JA (1990) Treatment of arteriovenous malformations of the brain with combined embolization and stereotactic radiosurgery: results after 1 and 2 years. AJNR 11: 857–864

2. Hirsch A, Norén G (1988) Audiological findings after stereotactic radiosurgery in acoustic neurinomas. Acta Otolaryngol (Stockh) 106: 244–251

3. Kemeny AA, Dias PS, Forster DMC (1989) Results of stereotactic radiosurgery of arteriovenous malformations: an analysis of 52 cases. J Neurol Neurosurg Psychiatry 52: 554–558

4. Kondziolka D, Lunsford LD, Coffey RJ, Bissonette DJ, Flickinger JC (1990) Stereotactic radiosurgery of angiographically occult vascular malformations: indications and preliminary experience. Neurosurgery 27: 892–900

5. Leksell L, Leksell D, Schwebel J (1985) Stereotaxis and nuclear magnetic resonance. Technical note. J Neurol Neurosurg Psychiatry 48: 14–18

6. Lindquist C, Steiner L (1988) Stereotactic radiosurgical treatment of arteriovenous malformations. In: Lunsford LD (ed) Modern stereotactic neurosurgery. Martinus Nijhoff, Boston, pp 491–505

7. Lobato RD, Perez C, Rivas JJ, Cordobes F (1988) Clinical, radiological, and pathological spectrum of angiographically occult intracranial vascular malformations. Analysis of 21 cases and review of the literature. J Neurosurg 68: 518–531

8. Lunsford LD, Kondziolka D, Flickinger JC, Bissonette DJ, Jungreis CA, Maitz AH, Horton JA, Coffey RJ (1991) Stereotactic radiosurgery of arteriovenous malformations of the brain. J Neurosurg 75: 512–524

9. Sadler LR, Jungreis CA, Lunsford LD, Trapanotto MM (1990) Angiographic technique to precede gamma knife radiosurgery for intracranial arteriovenous malformations. AJNR 11: 1157–1161

10. Spiegelmann R, Friedman WA, Bova FJ (1992) Limitations of angiographic target localization in planning radiosurgical treatment. Neurosurgery 30: 619–624

11. Steiner L, Leksell L, Greitz T, Forster DMC, Backlund EO (1972) Stereotaxic radiosurgery for cerebral arteriovenous malformations. Report of a case. Acta Chir Scand 138: 459–464

12. Stephanian E, Lunsford LD, Coffey RJ, Bissonette DJ, Flickinger JC (1992) Gamma knife surgery for sellar and suprasellar tumors. Neurosurg Clin North Am 3: 207–218

Correspondence: E. Schindler, M.D., Department of Diagnostic Radiology, Division of Neuroradiology, University of Vienna Medical School, Währinger Gürtel 18–20, A – 1090 Wien, Austria.

Acta Neurochir (1995) [Suppl] 63: 16–19

CT-Guided Needle Biopsy of Intracranial Tumours: Results in 118 Consecutive Patients

J. Duquesnel, F. Turjman, M. Hermier, Y. Bascoulergue, A. Jouvet, G. Gervesy, and **P. Tournut**

Service de Radiologie, Hôpital Neurologique et Neurochirurgical "Pierre Wertheimer", Lyon, France

Summary

The purpose of this paper is to evaluate the efficacy and safety of CT-guided needle biopsies and to determine the optimal indications for this technique. The case histories of 118 patients who underwent a CT-guided biopsy for brain lesions during a six-year period, from Novermber 1986 to September 1992, were reviewed. During a preliminary CT-scan, the entry site was determined and localized using a radio opaque marker and the safest route to the lesion was chosen. One hundred and thirty four procedures were performed in 118 patients. A positive diagnosis of tumour was obtained in 106 patients (89.8%). Repeat procedures were required in 18 patients. High-grade gliomas were the more common lesions (55.1%). Morbidity and mortality was assessed over the 30-day period after the procedure. Nine patients died during this time. Eight patients from day 3 to day 30 in the expected course of their disease and one within 48 first hours from neurological deterioration following the procedure. We found that CT-scan guided biopsies are a safe and accurate way to obtain brain tissue specimens for pathological diagnosis in selected cases. For superficial and large tumours it is a simple, fast and effective procedure.

Keywords: Brain tumour; CT-guided biopsy; pathological diagnosis.

Introduction

Pathological verification is required prior to brain tumour treatment. Radiological findings are not sufficient to determine the best therapeutic management. Non-tumoural lesions–such as abscesses or old haematomas–can mimick brain tumours and need to be identified. The current technique of choice in brain tumours identification is the stereotactical biopsy. Based upon our experience in the treatment of brain abscesses using CT-guided technique, we performed CT-guided needle biopsies for selected brain tumours since 1986. The purpose of this paper is to evaluate the efficacy and safety of this procedure performed in 118 patients, and to determine the optimal indications for this technique.

Material and Methods

Characteristics of Population

The case histories of all patients who underwent a CT-guided biopsy for brain lesions during a six-year period from November 1986 to September 1992 were reviewed. Patients with non-tumoural lesions were excluded. One hundred and eighteen patients were included. They were 81 males and 37 females (sex ratio 2:2/1). Patients ranged in age from nine months to 82 years, with a mean age of 56.8 years. A relevant medical history was noted in 27 cases: in 23 patients, a prior history of neoplasm, either cerebral or extracerebral, was found: tuberculosis antecedents and AIDS were noted in three patients and a single case respectively. Delay between the onset of clinical symptoms and first procedure was less than one month in 52.2% of cases, between one and six months in 46.1%, between six and 12 months and more than 12 months in 0.85% each. The characteristics of tumours (number of lesions, site, and size) are summarized in Tables 1–3.

Description of the Technique

The procedure is first discussed by a neurosurgeon and a neuro-radiologist. The safest route to the lesion is chosen. During a preliminary CT-scan, the entry site is determined and localized using a radio opaque marker. A burr hole is surgically sited. The patient is then positioned in the CT-scanner. A side hole is made in the plastic catheter of the biopsy needle, a n° 14 angiocath. Under sterile conditions and local anaesthesia, the needle is introduced into the brain, toward the lesion. One or several CT-scan controls are usually performed during the needle progression. Once the catheter is inside the target lesion, the needle is removed (Figs. 1 and 2). The biopsy is taken by aspiration through the catheter. This biopsy is immediately analyzed, and when necessary a second biopsy is performed. One or

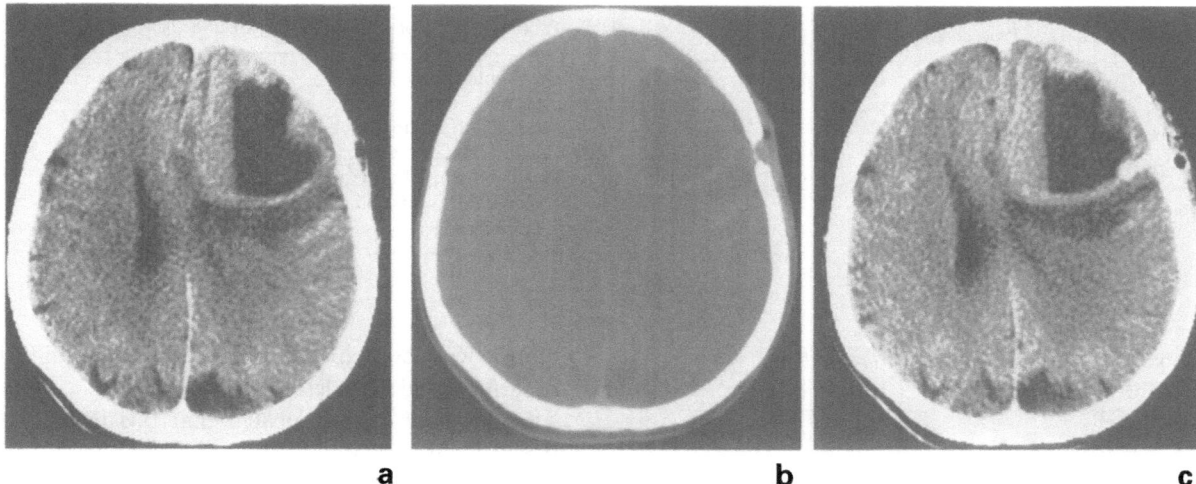

a   **b**   **c**

Fig. 1. (a) CT-scan with enhancement showing a large left heterogeneous frontal mass. (b) A burr-hole is done at the side (in front) of the lesion. (c) The plastic biopsy catheter is positioned at the margin of the lesion

several biopsies performed the same day are called "one procedure". A CT-scan is obtained immediately following the procedure to evaluate haemorrhagic complications.

Results

One hundred and thirty four procedures were performed in 118 patients. A positive diagnosis of tumour was obtained in 106 patients (89.8%). Repeat pro-

Table 1. *Number of Intracranial Lesions at CT Scan*

1 Lesion	80 patients	(67.8%)
2 Lesions	22 patients	(18.6%)
3 Lesions	12 patients	(10.2%)
More than 3	4 patients	(3.4%)

Table 2. *Location of Biopsied Tumours*

Frontal lobe	21
Parietal lobe	44
Occipital lobe	16
Temporal lobe	28
Thalamus	2
Corpus callosum	6
Suprasellar	1

Table 3. *Size of the Lesions*

Less than 2 cm	3.5%
2–4 cm	62%
4–6 cm	31%
More than 6 cm	3.5%

cedures were required in 18 patients (Table 4). High-grade gliomas were the more common lesions (55.1%). Other tumours included medium and low grade gliomas, metastasis, lymphoma, oligodendroglioma, PNET, meningioma and craniopharyngioma (Table 5). In 10 cases, a complementary surgical biopsy was taken. In 5 cases, the diagnosis was confirmed. In 3 cases, the diagnosis was different after surgical biopsy: a craniopharyngioma became an optic nerve glioma, a grade I or II astrocytoma became a grade III astrocytoma and a grade II astrocytoma became a grade IV astrocytoma. In two cases, surgical biopsies were positive after negative CT-guided biopsies.

Morbidity and mortality was assessed over the 30-day period after the procedure. Nine patients died

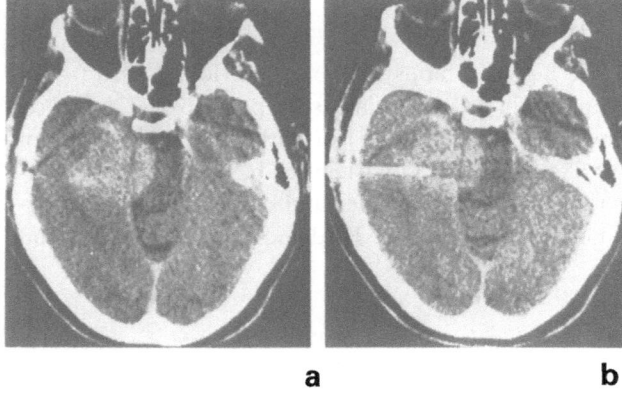

a   **b**

Fig. 2. (a) CT-scan with enhancement shows a large right temporal mass. (b) A biopsy needle was passed through a burr hole. The pathological diagnosis was grade III astrocytoma

Table 4. *Number of Procedures (n = 134)*

	One	Two	Three
Patients with positive diagnosis of tumour	92 (78%)	13 (11%)	1 (8.5%)
Patients with negative diagnosis of tumour	8 (6.8%)	4 (3.4%)	0

Table 7. *Results of Immediate Check CT-Scan*

No modification	81 patients
Presence of air	7 patients
Minimal intratumoural blood trace	22 patients
Parenchymal haematoma	13 patients
Small extradural haematoma	1 patient
Minimal intraventricular haemorrhage	1 patient

Table 5. *Histological Diagnosis Provided by CT-Guided Biopsies*

	Number of patients
Craniopharyngioma	1
Meningioma	1
PNET	2
Oligodendroglioma	4
Lymphoma	5
No diagnosis	12
Metastasis	14
Astrocytoma grade I & II	14
Astrocytoma grade III & IV	65

during this time. Eight patients from day 3 to day 30 in the expected course of their disease and one within 48 hours from first neurological deterioration following the procedure. Table 6 summarizes the pathological findings in these nine patients. No modifications occurred in 83% of patients (n = 98). Neurological impairment was noted in 8 patients (6.8%) and was transitory in 3 and permanent in 5 (4.2%).

Results of an immediate check CT-scan are summarized in Table 7.

Discussion

CT-guided biopsy has been previously used to obtain brain tissue specimens for pathological diagnosis without [5, 8, 11, 15, 17] or with [6, 12, 13] the use of a fixation frame. Goldstein [5] has reported a comparison between CT-guided and stereotaxic cranial diagnostic needle biopsies. He demonstrated that free hand

Table 6. *Histologic Diagnosis in Patients Deceased During the 30 Day Period*

Grade III and IV astrocytoma	7/9 (77.8%)
Metastasis	1/9 (11.1%)
Lymphoma	1/9 (11.1%)

biopsy was less expensive and time consuming for superficial and large lesions.

Coffey *et al.* [4] advocated that this technique is theoretically more likely to complicate than a stereotaxic procedure. They considered that free hand biopsy necessitates trajectory adjustment that traumatizes the brain overlying the lesion. The lack of a fixation device risks a leucotomy effect. In case of repeated biopsies during the same procedure, the CT-guidance does not allow exactly the same route toward the lesion. In our experience, the risk of a CT-guided procedure was comparable to the risk of the stereotactic procedures as reported in the literature. The complications related to our procedures included one death (0.84%) and 5 cases of permanent neurological impairment (4.2%). Recent stereotaxic series presented a 1.4% mortality rate and 5.7% morbidity rate [1, 3, 7, 9, 10, 14]. We need to emphasize that the populations of both techniques are not the same, especially when considering the size and location of the tumour. In consequence, the comparison of the two techniques is not completely valid. Our low rate of complications shows that CT-guided procedures may be considered as safe. This confirms the experience of the CT-guided brain abscess aspiration technique [2].

Haemorrhagic events were found in 15 out of 118 patients and were mostly asymptomatic. Since check CT-scans were routine, these patients were carefully monitored in association with the neuro-surgical team.

This procedure has to be safe but also effective. In our experience the pathological diagnosis was obtained in 89.8% of cases. These results are acceptable when compared with the diagnostic success rate of other reported series, ranging from 75% to 96% in the stereotactic series [1, 3, 7, 9, 10] and from 78% to 97% in the free-hand biopsies series [5, 6, 8, 11, 13, 15, 17]. There is a difference in the precision of the needle placement with both techniques. Stereotaxic biopsy is reported to be accurate within 1 mm. This advantage is important in the case of small lesions or small targets inside the lesion. We usually limited our technique to lesions larger than 2 cm in diameter. In fact most of the lesions encountered were large and easy to reach.

In three cases, the pathological results after surgical biopsies were different from percutaneous CT-guided biopsies. These cases are interesting and must be developed. At the beginning of our experience, a nine month old child suffered cardiac arrest during the craniotomy performed for the surgical removal of a suprasellar mass. A CT-guided biopsy was performed through the craniotomy and the pathological diagnosis was craniopharyngioma based upon the presence of keratinocytes. Further surgical exploration and biopsy demonstrated an optic glioma. The mistake was due to skin fragments taken with the specimen during the biopsy. In two other cases, the tumoural grade was underestimated; this was probably due to the biopsy procedure itself and is probably not dependent on the guiding technique.

As previous authors, we found that CT-scan is a safe and accurate way to obtain brain tissue specimens for pathological diagnosis. For superficial and large tumours, it is a simple, fast and effective procedure. We believe that the precision of a stereotactic approach is not required for these large lesions and that the risk of a non-fixed needle is probably theoretical.

References

1. Apuzzo MLJ, Sabshin JK (1983) Computed tomographic guidance stereotaxis in the management of intracranial mass lesions. Neurosurgery 12: 277–285
2. Bidzinski J, Koszewski W (1990) The value of different methods of treatment of brain abscess in the CT. Acta Neurochir (Wien) 105: 117–120
3. Bouvier G, Gouillard P, Leger SL *et al* (1983) Stereotactic biopsy of cerebral space-occupying lesions. Appl Neurophysiol 46: 227–230
4. Coffey RJ, Lunsford LD (1988) Reply to J. Goldstein *et al* J Neurosurg 68: 655–656
5. Goldstein S, Gumerlock MK, Neuwelt EA (1987) Comparison of CT-guided and stereotaxic cranial diagnostic needle biopsies. J Neurosurg 67: 341–347
6. Greenblatt SH, Rayport M, Savolaine ER *et al* (1982) Computed tomography-guided intracranial biopsy and cyst aspiration. Neurosurgery 11: 589–598
7. Heilbrun MP, Roberts TS, Apuzzo MLJ *et al* (1983) Preliminary experience with Brown-Roberts-Wells (BRW) computerized tomography stereotaxic guidance system. J Neurosurg 59:217–222
8. James HE, Wells M, Alksne JF *et al* (1979) Needle biopsy under computerized tomographic control: a method for tissue diagnosis in intracranial lesions. Neurosurgery 5: 671–674
9. Lobato RD, Rivas JJ, Cabello A *et al* (1982) Stereotactic biopsy of brain lesions visualized with computed tomography. Appl Neurophysiol 45: 426–430
10. Lunsford LD, Martinez AJ (1984) Stereotactic exploration of the brain in the era of computed tomography. Surg Neurol 22: 222–230
11. Maroon JC, Bank WO, Drayer BP *et al* (1977) Intracranial biopsy assisted by computerized tomography. J Neurosurg 46: 740–744
12. Moran CJ, Naidich TP, Gado MH *et al* (1979) Central nervous system lesions biopsied or treated by CT-guided needle placement. Radiology 131: 681–686
13. Moran CJ, Naidich TP, Marchoski JA (1984) CT-guided needle placement in the central nervous system: results in 146 consecutive patients. AJR 143: 861–868
14. Ostertag CB, Mennel HD, Kiessling M (1980) Stereotactic biopsy of brain tumors. Surg Neurol 14: 275–283
15. Rushworth RG (1980) Stereotactic guided biopsy in the computerized tomography scanner. Surg Neurol 14: 451–454
16. Savitz MH, Katz SS, Jimenez JP *et al* (1983) Biopsy and drainage of intracerebral lesions by CT-guided needle. Mt Sinai J Med 50: 326–330
17. Yeates A, Enzmann DR, Britt RH *et al* (1982) Simplified and accurate CT-guided needle biopsy of central nervous system lesions. J Neurosurg 57: 390–393

Correspondence: Francis Turjman, M.O., Hôpital Neurologique, Service de Radiologie, 59, Boulevard Pinel, 69003 Lyon, France.

Acta Neurochir (1995) [Suppl] 63: 20–24

The Role of Stereotactic Biopsy in Radiosurgery

F. Alesch[1], J. Pappaterra[1], S. Trattnig[2], and W. Th. Koos[1]

[1]Neurochirurgische Universitätsklinik and [2]Institut für Magnetresonanz, Wien, Austria

Summary

Radiosurgery offers a very powerful, minimally invasive therapeutic tool in the modern treatment of intracranial lesions. A direct contact with the lesion, as always takes place, e.g. in a stereotactic biopsy or microsurgical operation, is no longer an absolute prerequisite. Treatment planning is done using modern imaging techniques like computer assisted tomography (CT) or magnetic resonance imaging (MRI). Both provide high resolution and contrast images. The lesions can be displayed with high accuracy. The specificity of these techniques is adequate enough to provide neuropathological data which are a prerequisite for treatment?

In 1991 we published a retrospective study in which the diagnosis based on CT was compared with the histological diagnosis following stereotactic biopsy on a series of 181 patients with intracranial processes. We could show clearly that CT alone does not offer a reliable basis for therapy planning. Overall CT-scan was inaccurate in 22% of the cases.

Now in an additional series of 195 patients with intracranial processes, we have compared the MRI diagnosis with the neuropathological diagnosis.

MRI results and the neuropathological diagnosis based on microsurgical operation were compared and evaluated according to the following criteria:
1. Absolute agreement between MRI and histological diagnosis.
2. No agreement between MRI and histological diagnosis.
3. Conditional agreement: the MRI result offered several differential diagnoses one of which was accurate.

The highest rate of accurate diagnoses was seen in non-glial tumours with 78% correct 10% wrong and 12% conditionally agreeing diagnoses. In this category, pituitary adenomas reached even 90%. The results were poor in gliomas (33, 28, 39%) and in non-neoplastic lesions (30, 40, 30%). In sharply demarcated lesions and in those located in the area of the skull base, the diagnostic accuracy was significantly better than in other lesions. Compared to CT, the diagnostic accuracy of MRI seems to be significantly superior in non-glial tumours, while it is inferior in glial tumours.

As a conclusion we feel that, even in view of the greater accuracy of MRI over CT; it cannot replace the neuropathological examination, which can only takes place under the microscope.

Keywords: Stereotaxy; MRI; CT; reliability; histology; radiosurgery.

Introduction

The advances in the field of computer-assisted imaging like computer assisted tomography (CT) and magnetic resonance imaging (MRI) in the last two decades have led to considerable improvement in the diagnostics of intracranial processes. Even the smallest lesions can be clearly represented and are thus often discovered before they lead to symptoms. Parallel to this development in diagnosis, the quality of therapeutic procedures has also improved. The primary aim of this improvement is the minimisation of the invasiveness of operations with a simultaneous increase in their efficiency. Radiosurgery plays an important role in this development. This technique, also known as stereotactic convergent beam irradiation, permits the treatment of intracranial processes without opening of the cranium. The therapy planning is based only on CT or MRI. This means that direct contact as it always takes place, e.g. in a microsurgical operation, is no longer an absolute prerequisite for treatment.

However, this method considerably increases the significance of the following problem: Is the specificity of modern imaging diagnosis such as CT-scan or MRI sufficiently accurate that it can form the basis for definitive therapeutic measures? The high sensitivity of both procedures has already been mentioned above. The question of whether their reliability is sufficient to replace neuropathological examination, such as is carried out on stereotactically or microsurgically obtained biopsy material, remains open.

In 1991 we published a retrospective study in which the diagnosis based on CT was compared with the histological diagnosis following stereotactic biopsy on a series of 181 patients with intracranial processes [1, 2].

The results of our study at that time clearly indicated that CT alone does not offer a reliable basis for treatment planning. Based on the fact that the histopathological diagnosis expressed in the CT-scan was inaccurate in 22% of the cases in our series, we concluded that CT cannot replace neuropathological examination.

However, the article published in 1991 was based solely on CT-diagnostics. MRI was not taken into consideration as an additional computer-assisted diagnostic procedure. Therefore, the question of whether MRI diagnosis could possibly replace a neuropathological examination remained open.

Referring back to our CT study, we have compared the MRI diagnosis with the neuropathological diagnosis in an additional series of 195 patients with intracranial processes. In contrast to the CT series this study does not involve cases of stereotactic biopsies, but rather microsurgical operations.

Method

All of the 195 patients included in this study had been examined by MRI at the Institute for Magnetic Resonance at the University of Vienna. The examinations were performed either on a 1.5 T imaging system* or a 0.5 T unit** using a circular polarised head coil. Axial T2-weighted stand TSE-sequences and axial, coronal and optional sagittal T1-weighted SE-sequences before and after i.v. administration of 0.2 ml/kg body weight Gadolinium-DTPA*** were performed. Sometimes a T1-weighted 3D gradient echo-sequence (MP-RAGE and T1-Volume FFE, respectively) was applied after administration of contrast media. Slice thickness and gap varied from 6/06, to 3/0 and 1.5 min 3D-sequences.

Thereafter all patients were subjected to neurosurgical treatment. The samples of the lesions were examined as smear preparations, and also after fixation and paraffin embedding. If there was a need immunohistochemical methods were carried out. The results of the neuropathological examination are given in Table 2.

The MRI diagnoses used for this study were based solely on the pre-operative written results. In addition, the following criteria were taken into consideration: localisation, size, contrast medium enhancement, number of lesions, perifocal oedema and resolution with respect to the surrounding area.

The diagnosis based on the MRI result and the histological diagnosis based on the microsurgical operation were compared and evaluated according to the following criteria (Table 3):

1. Absolute agreement between MRI and histological diagnosis (group 1).
2. No agreement between MRI and histological diagnosis (group 2).
3. Conditional agreement: the MRI result offered several differential diagnoses, one of which was accurate (group 3).

---

* SP 4000, Siemens, Erlangen, Germany.
** Gyroscan T5, Philips, Eindhoven, The Netherlands.
*** Magnevist, Schering, Berlin, Germany.

Table 1. *Accuracy of the CT and MRI Diagnoses in the Different Categories of Neuropathological Diagnoses (see Table 2).* The diagnosis based on these imaging techniques and the corresponding neuropathological diagnosis were compared and evaluated according to the following critera: agreement, no agreement, conditional agreement. Statistical significance was calculated to detect differences between CT and MRI diagnostic accuracy

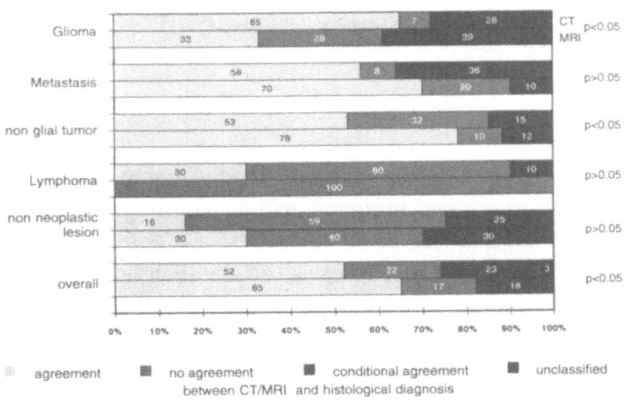

CT:n = 181, MRI:n = 195.

Table 2. *Neuropathological Diagnoses after Smear Preparation and Paraffin Section (n = 195)*

	n
Glial tumours:	
Low grade astrocytoma	18
High grade astrocytoma	3
Ependymoma	5
Oligodendroglioma	4
Glioblastoma	9
Metastases:	10
Lymphoma:	1
Non-glial tumours:	
Pituitary adenoma	42
Meningioma	42
Neurinoma	18
Craniopharyngioma	4
Epidermoid	4
Hemangioma	4
Medulloblastoma	4
Chordoma	3
Chondroma	2
Germinoma	2
Colloid cyst	2
Malignant tumour	2
Gangliocytoma	1
Benign tumour	1
Non-neoplastic lesions:	
Cavernoma	4
Infection	3
Haematoma	2
Abscess	1
No classification possible:	4

22

Table 3. *The MRI Results were Compared to the Histological Result and Classified in the Following Groups*

Group 1	Agreement between the MRI and histological diagnoses.
Group 2	No agreement between the MRI and histological diagnoses.
Group 3	The histological diagnosis did appear in the MRI result, but under several possible differential diagnoses, so that ambiguity was not resolved until the operation.

Results

The histopathological diagnoses according to examination of the smear preparation and paraffin embedding are summarised in Table 2.

In analogy to our CT-series the classification was done according to the following histological categories: glial tumours ($n = 39$), metastases ($n = 10$), lymphomas ($n = 1$), non-glial tumours ($n = 131$) and non-neoplastic lesions ($n = 10$). In 4 cases a neuropathological classification was not possible.

A comparison of the MRI diagnoses with the histological diagnoses according to the criteria in Table 3 showed that the diagnostic accuracy of MRI for the gliomas was 33% (group 1). In 28% the MRI diagnosis was incorrect (group 2) and in 39% it was ambiguous (group 3). For the metastases the ratio was 70, 20, 10%; for the non-glial tumours 78, 10, 12%. The only lymphoma in our series was incorrectly diagnosed. However, in order to allow a comparability with the CT series it was included in its own category. The accuracy for the non-neoplastic lesions was 30, 40, 30%. In relation to the entire series the accuracy was 65, 17, 18%.

In the region of the cranial base MRI provides artefact-free images with high resolution and therefore is superior to CT. This explains why processes in this area were represented with overproportional frequency: 42 pituitary adenomas, 42 meningiomas, 18 neurinomas and 4 craniopharyngeomas. These processes will be displayed and discussed separately:

The diagnostic accuracy of MRI was highest for pituitary adenomas at 90%. In 5% the diagnosis was incorrect; in another 5% it was ambiguous. For the meningiomas the ratio was 86, 5, 9%. There were no inaccurate diagnoses for the neurinomas; however, possible differential diagnoses were considered in 22%, one of which then proved to be accurate. The diagnostic accuracy for the craniopharyngeomas was notably poorer at 50%. In the remaining 50% the MRI diagnosis was incorrect.

The overall accuracy in this category was 84% with 6% errors and 10% ambiguous diagnoses. These results are given in Table 4.

For the group of incorrectly diagnosed cases (group 2) we have contrasted histological and MRI diagnoses separately and then correlated them (Table 5). These results are examined in more detail in the Discussion section.

In searching for possible causes of diagnostic errors we have established correlations between the parameters listed in Table 6 and the diagnostic accuracy. For the parameters "boundary to the surrounding area" and "localisation" there was a significant difference. The diagnostic accuracy was higher in sharper delineated lesions and in those located in the area of the skull base. Pituitary adenomas, neurinomas and meningiomas fulfil these criteria and were, as already mentioned, numerically greater in our series. The other parameters (size, contrast medium enhancement, number of lesions, perifocal oedema) appear to have no influence on the accuracy.

We then compared the accuracy of the MRI series with that of the earlier CT series. In order to make such a comparison possible, the same categories were used.

Statistically significant differences appeared for all categories except for the metastases. The overall difference was also significant (Table 1). For the gliomas, lymphomas and non-neoplastic lesions, the diagnostic accuracy of MRI was inferior to CT. In contrast in non-glial tumours and overall the MRI accuracy was higher.

Table 4. *Accuracy of MRI Diagnosis in the Most Frequent Neuropathological Entities of Our Series.* These are mainly non-glial tumours of the cranial base, where MRI provides artefact-free images with high resolution and therefore is superior to CT. Evaluation was done according to criteria of Table 3

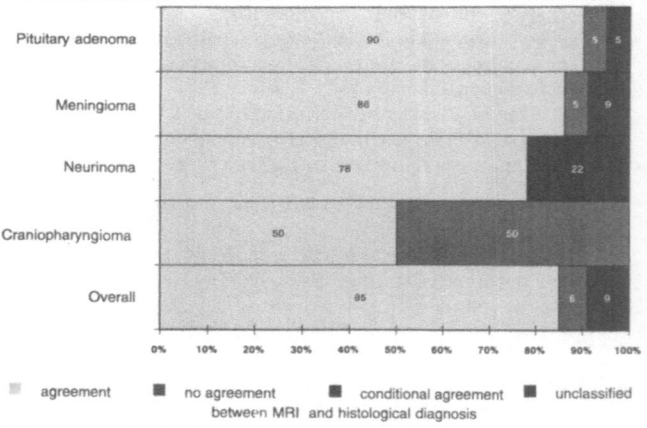

MRI: n = 106.

Table 5. *Juxtaposition of MRI and Histological Diagnoses for the Group of Incorrectly Diagnosed Cases.* Lymphomas and meningiomas were presumed several times in MRI and could not be verified histologically

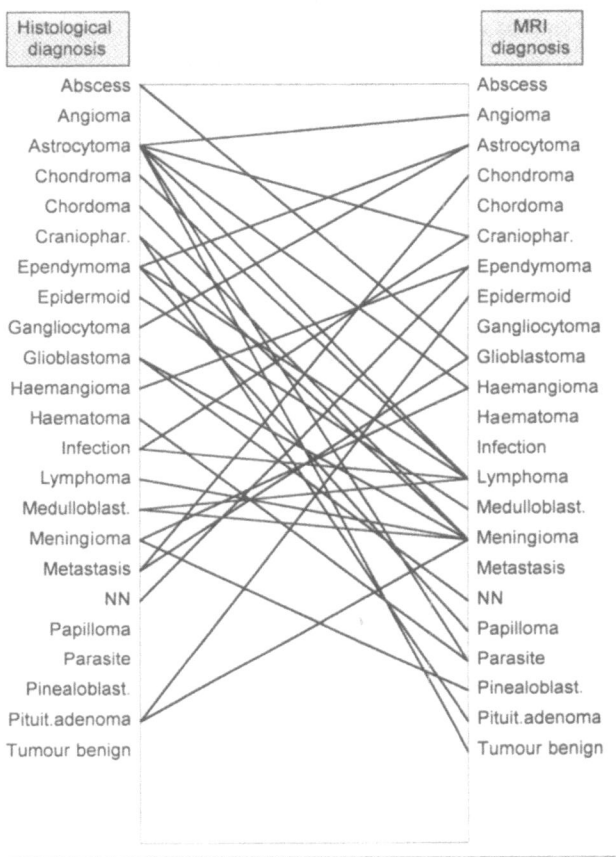

Table 6. *Criteria Included in the Evaluation of the MRI Result*

Localisation of the lesion:	
cortical:	27
subcortical:	43
basal ganglia:	3
cerebellum:	4
pons, vermis	60
sella, suprasellar, cranial base	58
Size of the lesion:	
<2 cm:	40
2–4 cm:	102
>4 cm:	53
Contrast medium enhancement:	
yes:	195
no:	0
Number of lesions:	
1:	182
2:	9
>2:	4
Perifocal edema:	
yes:	119
no:	76
Boundary to the surrounding area:	
sharp:	112
not sharp:	83

Discussion

Improvements in the quality of MRI and CT increase the contrast and the plasticity of the images. Topography is represented with a higher resolution. Even changes of a few millimetres in diameter can be detected. Unfortunately, this improvement in quality misleads one to confuse localisation, form and extension of a lesion with its histology. We often forget that these methods provide only physical information. As a rule these are only secondary changes such as necroses, oedema or alterations of the blood-brain barrier. Only different signal characteristics or density values are measured; they are then represented as hypo-, iso- or hyperintense respectively hypo-, iso- or hyperdense areas. However, there are no reliable standard values or (appearance) images, which for example would be accurate only for one type of tumour [2, 3].

Based on a series of 181 cases we were able to demonstrate that CT cannot provide any reliable infor-

mation on the histological nature of a lesion. However, such information is necessary before treatment is planned. In the series in question, MRI diagnoses were compared with neuropathological diagnoses. It was shown that the overall accuracy of MRI is superior to that of CT. We attribute this higher accuracy primarily to the numerical predominance of the processes in the region of the cranial base (sella, clivus, cerebello-pontine angle). In this region MRI is notably superior to CT since there are practically no bone artefacts thus increasing resolution. This implies that for the series, as compared to our previously published CT series, processes such as pituitary adenomas, meningiomas and neurinomas were relatively numerically predominant. The diagnosis for these processes is based not only on their morphology; the topography likewise plays an important role. This accounts for the fact that in a high percentage the MRI-based diagnosis was accurate for these histological entities. The diagnostic accuracy for gliomas is notably poorer and is thus also significantly below that of CT. On the other hand, it is higher, but not significantly so, for metastases. The relatively high agreement ratio as well in CT as in MRI can be explained by the fact that these processes usually have a characteristic spherical form and often appear in multiples. Several foci were present in 4 of our 10 metastases cases; not one was incorrectly diagnosed.

A particularly low accuracy for the lymphomas was observed in the CT series. We attributed this to the fact that they belong to the somewhat rarer neoplasms of the brain and are thus correspondingly rarely considered in differential diagnosis. In order to make a comparison with the CT series possible, we have included the only lymphoma in the MRI series separately. It was not detected. In contrast it was shown, as it can be seen in Table 5, that the lymphoma diagnosis was presumed several times on MRI and could not be verified by the neuropathological examination.

The non-neoplastic processes represent a very heterogeneous group. For this reason, but also because of the low number of patients with such processes, we can only draw speculative conclusions. This applies to the individual groups per se and also the comparison with CT. It is worth mentioning that in this series, 3 of the 4 cavernomas were diagnosed accurately and one was diagnosed conditionally.

In our series we were able to show that the accuracy for lesions with a high boundary to the environment is statistically significantly higher than for lesions with a poor one. Here we see a direct connection with the readily diagnosable processes of the cranial base.

This study is strictly retrospective and is based only on the written evaluation of the results. Use of the MRI images for the group classification was intentionally avoided in order to prevent a subsequent undesired adjustment of the results. An additional problem lies in the fact that the random sampling is very heterogeneous with respect to both the number and the diagnoses. It was therefore not an aim of our research to provide absolute numbers on the reliability of modern computer-assisted imaging diagnoses. This topic remains for a prospective study. On the contrary, it was shown that considerable residual inaccuracy remains, a fact that must be taken into account before invasive therapeutic steps are taken. Although a MRI diagnosis appears to be overall superior to a CT diagnosis with respect to accuracy, it cannot replace the neuropathological examination, which can only be performed with tissue samples under the microscope.

Acknowledgements

The neuropathological evaluation was done by H. Budka, Neurological Institute, University of Vienna.

References

1. Alesch F, Ostertag C, Dietrich B, Piepgras U (1991) Korrelation computertomographischer Befunde mit histologischen Diagnosen. Akt Neurol 18: 95–9
2. Dietrich B, Alesch F (1989) Specificity of CT diagnosis assessed by stereotaxic brain biopsy. A retrospective analysis of 180 cases. In: Nadjimi M (eds) Imaging of brain metabolism, spine and cord, interventional neuroradiology. Springer, Berlin Heidelberg New York Tokyo
3. Friedman WA, Sceats DJ, Nestok BR, Ballinger WE (1989) The incidence of unexpected pathological findings in an image-guided biopsy series: a review of 100 consecutive cases. Neurosurgery 25: 180–4
4. Mundinger F, Weigel K, Fürmaier R, Volk B (eds) (1986) CT and MRI diagnoses of intracranial tumours compared with the results of stereotactic biopsy. Springer, Berlin Heidelberg New York Tokyo

Correspondence: François Alesch, M.D., Neurochirurgische Universitätsklinik, Währinger Gürtel 18–20, A-1090 Wien, Austria.

Acta Neurochir (1995) [Suppl] 63: 25–28

Indications for Brachytherapy for Brain Tumours

M. Bernstein and **N. Laperriere**

Division of Neurosurgery, The Toronto Hospital and Department of Radiation Oncology, Princess Margaret Hospital, University of Toronto, Toronto, Ontario, Canada

Summary

The authors summarize the indications for brachytherapy for brain tumours based on the available data from the literature and on general principles relating to the radiobiology of brachytherapy and the natural biology of brain tumours.

Keywords: Brachytherapy; brain tumours; indications.

Introduction

Brachytherapy is a powerful focal therapy for both the palliative and curative treatment of various solid tumours [21, 24] and has been used for brain neoplasms for 80 years [2]. However, the modern age of brachytherapy dawned when sophisticated dosimetry could be combined with precise image-guided placement of radiation sources using stereotactic surgery married to accurate imaging (i.e. computed tomography initially and subsequently magnetic resonance imaging). In spite of the physical and mathematical accuracy of brachytherapy, this modality has largely been applied in non-randomized studies and relatively little is known about its efficacy for patients with brain tumours. Only two randomized studies have been conceived (both for newly diagnosed patients with malignant astrocytoma), and both are nearing completion [4]. Non-randomized studies have examined the use of brachytherapy for de novo malignant astrocytoma [4, 19], recurrent malignant astrocytoma [4, 15], de novo low-grade astrocytoma [9, 16], de novo and recurrent metastases [12, 20], and de novo and recurrent extra-axial skull base neoplasms [13, 14].

In this brief review, we examine the relative indications for interstitial brachytherapy for brain tumours;

intracystic therapy is not addressed herein. The conclusions and recommendations arrived at are based on available recorded clinical experience, radiobiological considerations, and our knowledge about the natural biology and response to conventional treatment of the various brain neoplasms presenting difficult treatment challenges to neuro-oncologists.

Malignant Astrocytoma: De novo Tumours

Since the outcome of patients treated conventionally for malignant astrocytoma (including glioblastoma multiforme) is so poor, experimental approaches are justified and needed. A radiation dose-response relationship exists for most cancer cells treated by experimental brachytherapy [3], and in humans, prospective randomized data may support a dose-response relationship regarding the radiotherapeutic treatment of these tumours [5]. Additionally, most recurrences occur within the initial treatment volume [1, 10] indicating that local control is the main challenge in the treatment of these tumours and that modalities directed at the initial tumour volume appear to be appropriate. The above statements summarize the rationale for brachytherapy as part of the initial treatment of malignant astrocytoma.

At present, because of the incontrovertible benefit of external radiation for these tumours [25] we feel that brachytherapy should be used as a "boost" following conventional therapy consisting of craniotomy or stereotactic biopsy followed by external fractionated radiation via regional fields to a dose of 50–60 Gy in 25–30 fractions, with or without concomitant chemotherapy. This scenario represents the situation for the bulk of the reported data on brachytherapy for de novo malignant astrocytoma [4, 15, 19]. Whether brachytherapy used in this way actually produces a statistically significant improvement in survival for patients with de novo malignant astrocytoma is not yet known but will be clarified by the two randomised studies nearing completion: the University of Toronto study and that of the Brain Tumour Cooperative Group [4]. If brachytherapy is to be used alone, that is without external radiation, then this must also initially be in the setting of an ethically and scientifically sound, randomized controlled study. In any case, it is clear that randomized studies are required to demonstrate differences between treatment groups since selection of patients alone can impact greatly on the outcome, irrespective of treatment given [8].

Patients with newly diagnosed supratentorial malignant astrocytoma should only be considered eligible for brachytherapy if they have good neurological and functional status (i.e. Karnofsky score should be 70 or better). The tumour (i.e. the enhancing edge) should be reasonably well demarcated on neurodiagnostic imaging (i.e. CT and/or MRI) and of maximum dimension 6 cm or less. Larger tumours are usually less well demarcated and also, larger volumes receiving high-dose radiation are more likely to produce neurological morbidity. Tumours producing significant mass effect should be reduced surgically prior to brachytherapy. Indistinct tumours are inappropriate because adequate dosimetric planning is not feasible if one cannot discern the borders of the enhancing portion of the tumour. The tumour should be unilateral and hemispheric; crossing of the midline in the corpus callosum and/or extension caudally into the upper brainstem are indicative of a less favourable tumour biology and also would be expected to result in high incidence of brachytherapy-induced morbidity. Tumours in eloquent locations such as dominant thalamus are technically eligible for brachytherapy but the risk of significant neurological deterioration is higher, and the opportunity for delayed reoperation which may be an integrally important part of brachytherapy regimes [4, 15, 19] will either be unfeasible and/or attendant with extremely high risk. Multicentric glioma should be excluded for a number of reasons, including the fact that there are certainly other microscopic lesions not seen on imaging which will not be treated and will portend a poor outcome for the patient. Finally, brachytherapy produces significant and prolonged cere-

bral edema in the majority of patients and the patient must not have a major contra-indication to protracted steroid use (e.g. active peptic ulcer). In the University of Toronto hospitals, only approximately 30% of patients with de novo malignant astrocytoma satisfy the above criteria and are eligible for brachytherapy.

Malignant Astrocytoma: Recurrent Tumours

Once a malignant astrocytoma recurs following conventional therapy, survivial is usually measurable in terms of months if no further therapy is given. Reoperation and chemotherapy offer modest prolongation of life in well-selected patients [6, 11] and brachytherapy has therefore been tried in this setting with modest but encouraging results [4, 15]. The indications for brachytherapy for patients with recurrent disease are similar to those for patients with de novo malignant astrocytoma. Tumour size should be 6 cm or less in maximum dimension, the recurrence should be solitary (i.e. not multicentric) and reasonably well-circumscribed, and not invading contralateral hemisphere or brainstem. Lesions productive of significant mass effect are likely to result in increased neurological deficit following brachytherapy and cyto-reductive surgery should be performed prior to consideration of brachytherapy in such patients. The patient's Karnofsky functional status should be at least 70 or better; patients with malignant brain tumours who are in poor neurological condition are well known to do relatively poorly from treatment (wether it be conventional or experimental) [7]. Patients who have had a reasonably long-relapse-free interval between their initial treatment and recurrence have been shown to benefit more from manoeuvres such as reoperation [6] and this likely suggests a slightly more favourable biology of their tumour; brachytherapy in such a patient would be expected to produce a very beneficial palliation. Of all patients with recurrent malignant astrocytoma evaluated at the University of Toronto hospitals, only about 10% fulfil the above criteria and are considered eligible for brachytherapy.

Low-Grade Astrocytoma

Brachytherapy has been used for supratentorial low-grade astrocytoma in Europe for decades [9, 16], but we feel there is no role for brachytherapy in this group of patients. In malignant astrocytoma, the benefit of external fractionated radiation has been incontrovertibly demonstrated in randomized studies to prolong survival [25]. The same cannot be said for low-grade astrocytoma. A number of retrospective reviews have arrived at conflicting results [18, 22, 23] but no prospective randomized study has been reported; a number of studies are underway or being conceived and the neuro-oncological community awaits the results of these studies with interest. At present, the biology of low-grade astrocytomas is sufficiently variable, and in some cases quite favourable, and many clinicians don't even treat them until clinical and/or radiological progression occurs. We feel that applying a potentially very toxic, unproven therapy to a disease with variable bilogy, often indistinct boundaries on imaging, and unproven response to conventional fractionated radiation is not scientifically sound.

Metastases

A modest experience with brachytherapy for de novo and recurrent brain metastases has been accrued [12, 20]. Since these tumours are histologically more circumscribed than gliomas, the rationale for their treatment with brachytherapy, or other focused radiation technique, is more compelling than for malignant astrocytoma. Best conventional treatment of a solitary brain metastasis consists of complete surgical resection if possible followed by external fractionated whole-brain radiation to doses ranging from 20 Gy in 5 fractions to 50 Gy in 25 fractions [17]. With this treatment the median survival is approximately 40 weeks [17] but some patients have long-term survival, or complete control of their brain tumour with death ensuing because of uncontrolled systemic disease. For this reason we feel that brachytherapy for de novo metastasis is unnecessary and potentially dangerous for the majority of patients with solitary brain metastasis amenable to surgical excision and external radiation. If brachytherapy is used for de novo metastasis, it must be combined with external fractionated whole-brain radiation because of the high incidence of multiplicity of metastatic deposits (either seen on MRI or microscopic). We feel the only justification for the current use of brachytherapy for de novo metastatic tumours would be as part of a properly designed randomized protocol.

We feel brachytherapy is most appropriate for brain metastases which recur following conventional therapy. The brain lesion must be solitary and within the cerebral hemisphere; cerebellar tumours are also eligible if they are not abutting the brainstem. The tumour should be less than 6 cm in maximum dimension and not associated with significant mass effect; if the latter situation obtains repeat craniotomy for removal of the tumour should be done prior to brachytherapy. Systemic disease must be under excellent control, that is in clinical and radiological remission. Again, the longer the patient has been recurrence-free following initial treatment, the more favourable the tumour's biology and the more likely is the patient to have a beneficial response to brachytherapy.

Skull Base Tumours

The data on brachytherapy for skull base tumours are few, but there is ample evidence that brachytherapy can have a radiologically measurable positive effect on both benign tumours (e.g. meningioma, pituitary adenoma) and malignant tumours (e.g. chordoma, chondrosarcoma) of the skull base [13, 14]. This modality has been used for de novo tumours in patients too old or infirm for radical surgery and for recurrent tumours where surgical and/or external radiation treatment has failed [13, 14]. There is too little data to draw conclusions or make treatment recommendations, but we can state that brachytherapy probably does have a small role to play in these tumours, and probably only in those cases where percutaneous stereotactic radiation cannot be used perhaps because of the anatomy and/or size of the lesion.

Conclusion

Brachytherapy, while a potent adjuvant therapy, has significant toxicity and unequivocal efficacy remains to be demonstrated for the common malignant brain tumours neuro-oncologists encounter. Patients must be well selected such that the maximum possible benefit accrues to those who are in a position to benefit from the therapy without incurring undue risk of morbidity. The results of two randomized studies are awaited, and further randomized studies will likely be required. Brachytherapy will probably continue to occupy an important role for highly selected patients with de novo and recurrent malignant astrocytoma, and for patients with recurrent solitary brain metastases which are too large for percutaneous stereotactic radiation.

References

1. Bashir R, Hochberg F, Oot R (1988) Regrowth patterns of glioblastoma multiforme related to planning of interstitial brachytherapy radiation fields. Neurosurgery 23: 27–30

2. Bernstein M, Gutin PH (1981) Interstitial brachytherapy for brain tumours: Review. Neurosurgery 9: 741–750

3. Bernstein M, Gutin PH, Weaver KA, Deen DF, Barcellos MH (1982) Iodine-125 interstitial implants in the RIF-1 murine flank tumour: an animal model for brachytherapy. Radiat Res 91: 624–637

4. Bernstein M, Laperriere N, Leung P, McKenzie S (1990) Interstitial brachytherapy for malignant brain tumours. Preliminary results. Neurosurgery 26: 371–380

5. Bleehen NM, Stenning SP (1991) A medical research council trial of two radiotherapy doses in the treatment of grades 3 and 4 astrocytoma. Br J Cancer 64: 769–774

6. Dirks P, Bernstein M, Muller PJ, Tucker WS (1993) The value of reoperation for recurrent glioblastoma. Can J Surg 36: 271–275

7. Duncan GG, Goodman GB, Ludgate CM, Rheaume DE (1992) The treatment of adult supratentorial high grade astrocytomas. J Neurooonc 13: 63–72

8. Florell RC, Macdonald DR, Irish WD, Bernstein M, Leibel SA, Gutin PH, Cairncross JG (1992) Selection bias, survival, and brachytherapy for glioma. J Neurosurg 76: 179–183

9. Frank F, Fabrizi AP, Frank-Ricci R, Sturiale C, Nuzzo G (1985) Treatment of low malignancy brain neoplasms by means of stereotactic interstitial radiotherapy. Appl Neurophysiol 48: 121–126

10. Hochberg FH, Pruitt (1980) Assumptions in the radiotherapy of glioblastoma. Neurology 30: 907–911

11. Kornblith PL, Walker M (1988) Chemotherapy for malignant gliomas. J Neurosurg 68: 1–17

12. Kreth FW, Warnke PC, Ostertag CB (1993) Stereotaktische interstitielle Radiochirurgie und perkutane Radiotherape in der Behandlung zerebraler Metastases. Nervenarzt 64: 108–113

13. Kumar PP, Good RG, Leibrock LG, Mawk JR, Yonkers AJ, Ogren FP (1988) High activity iodine 125 endocurietherapy for recurrent skull base tumours. Cancer 61: 1518–1527

14. Kumar PP, Patil AA, Leibrock LG, Chu W, Syh H, McCaul GF, Reeves MA (1993) Continuous low dose rate brachytherapy with high activity iodine-125 seeds in the management of meningiomas. Int J Rad Onc Biol Phys 25: 325–328

15. Leibel SA, Gutin PH, Wara WM, Silver PS, Larson DA, Edwards MSB, Lamb SA, Ham B, Weaver KA, Barnett C, Phillips TL (1989) Survival and quality of life after interstitial implantation of removable iodine-125 sources for the treatment of patients with recurrent malignant gliomas. Int J Rad Onc Biol Phys 17: 1129–1139

16. Mundinger F, Weigel K (1984) Indication and results of stereotactic curietherapy with iridium-192 and iodine-125 for non-resectable tumours of the hypothalamic region. Acta Neurochir (Wien) [Suppl] 33: 323–330

17. Patchell RA, Tibbs PA, Walsh JW, Dempsey RJ, Maruyama Y, Kryscio RJ, Markesbery WR, Mcdonald JS, Young B (1990) A randomized trial of surgery in the treatment of single metastases to the brain. N Engl J Med 322: 494–500

18. Philippon JH, Clemenceau SH, Fauchon FH, Foncin JF (1993) Supratentorial low-grade astrocytomas in adults. Neurosurgery 32: 554–559

19. Prados MD, Gutin PH, Phillips TL, Wara WM, Sneed PK, Larson DA, Lamb SA, Ham B, Malec MK, Wilson CB (1992) Interstitial brachytherapy for newly diagnosed patients with malignant gliomas: The UCSF experience. Int J Rad Onc Biol Phys 24: 593–597

20. Prados M, Leibel S, Barnett C, Gutin PH (1989) Interstitial brachytherapy for metastatic brain tumours. Cancer 63: 657–660

21. Raju PI, Roy T, McDonald RD, Harrison BR, Crim C, Hyers TM, Marshall SJ, Ohar JA, Naunheim KS (1993) IR-192 low dose-rate endobronchial brachytherapy in the treatment of malignant airway obstruction. Int J Rad Onc Biol Phys 27: 677–680

22. Recht LD, Lew R, Smith TW (1992) Suspected low-grade glioma: Is deferring treatment safe? Ann Neurol 31: 431–436

23. Shaw EG, Daumas-Duport C, Scheithauer BW, Gilbertson DT, O'Fallon JR, Earle JD, Laws ER, Okazaki H (1989) Radiation therapy in the management of low-grade supratentorial astrocytomas. J Neurosurg 70: 853–861

24. Vicini F, White J, Gustafson G, Matter RC, Clarke DH, Edmundson G, Martinez A (1993) The use of iodine-125 seeds as a substitute for iridium-192 seeds in temporary interstitial breast implants. Int J Rad Onc Biol Phys 27: 561–566

25. Walker MD, Alexander E, Hunt WE, MacCarty CS, Mahaley M, Mealey J, Norrell HA, Owens G, Ransohoff J, Wilson CB, Gehan EA, Strike TA (1978) Evaluation of BCNU and/or radiotherapy in the treatment of anaplastic gliomas. J Neurosurg 49: 333–343

Correspondence: Mark Bernstein, M.D., Division of Neurosurgery, The Toronto Hospital – Western Division, Suite 2-405, McLaughlin Pavilion, 399 Bathurst Street, Toronto, Ontario, M5T 2S8, Canada.

Acta Neurochir (1995) [Suppl] 63: 29–34

Interstitial Irradiation of Brain Metastases

F. Alesch[1], R. Hawliczek[2], and **W. Th. Koos**

[1]Neurochirurgische Universitätsklinik and [2]Universitätsklinik für Strahlentherapie und Strahlenbiologie, Wien, Austria

Summary

Randomized studies have shown that survival in patients with single brain metastases is significantly higher after the combined treatment of surgical removal and whole-brain irradiation than after whole-brain radiation therapy alone. In patients with deep-seated lesions or those located in critical sites of the brain, as well as in cases in which the patient's general condition makes general anaesthesia difficult or impossible microsurgical resection usually cannot be performed or only with an increased surgical risk. Stereotactic radiosurgery, which can be done by means of convergent beam irradiation or by the implantation of highly loaded ^{125}I seeds, provides an alternative to open procedures. In the following we report on our results using a stereotactic radiosurgical technique. A series of 20 treatments is presented, in which biopsy was performed and ^{125}I seeds were implanted, both under stereotactic conditions in the same session. The ^{125}I seeds were sealed in a teflon catheter, were left indwelling temporarily, and then removed after application of the prescribed radiation dose (6,000cGy at the tumour margin). There was only one recurrence in our series, complications occurred in only one patient by temporary aggravation of a pre-existing hemiparesis. Our results indicate that interstitial irradiation of brain metastases is a valuable, less stressful alternative to both open microsurgery as well as to stereotactic radiosurgical convergent beam irradiation.

Keywords: Stereotactic radiosurgery; brachycurietherapy; interstitial implant; metastases.

Introduction

The incidence of brain metastases has been increasing steadily over the last years [14, 15]. The reason for this is essentially unknown, however, one factor might be the progress made in palliative treatment (chemotherapy) of disseminated disease, which has resulted in more and more of these patients living long enough to develop brain metastases. Metastases are the most common malignant diseases of the brain, occurring more frequently than primary tumours such as gliomas. Symptomatic metastases occur in roughly 30% of patients with malignant disease and autopsy studies have revealed more than a 50% incidence [4, 18]. Untreated patients have a median survival of approximately one month, while patients receiving whole-brain radiotherapy have a median survival of three to six months [5, 10, 19]. Most patients ultimately die of systemic disease. The treatment of brain metastases in most cases is purely palliative.

There is a subgroup of patients, however, with only one single metastatic lesion in the brain and no further metastatic detectable malignant disease. A randomized study of these patients showed that the combination of surgical management plus postoperative whole-brain radiotherapy produced better results than whole-brain radiation alone [13, 16] in terms of survival and quality of life. Survival was significantly higher in the surgical group.

Despite the better results after surgery, the disadvantages associated with operation are the considerable strain produced by the anaesthesia and the prolonged hospitalisation, as well as the risk of postoperative neurologic deficits. In patients with deep-seated tumours or lesions located near critical structures of the brain, microsurgery is associated with increased surgical morbidity.

Stereotactic radiosurgery is an alternative to open surgery. The procedure can be used to treat deep-seated lesions and, since it requires only local anaesthesia, can be performed in patients whose general condition does not allow surgery under general anaesthesia. The goal of radiosurgery is to deliver a focused, high dose of radiation to the target volume, i.e. the metastasis, in order to provoke a local radionecrosis. This can be done in several ways: externally by means of stereotactic convergent beam irradiation (LINAC,

Gamma Unit) [6, 9, 17], or interstitially by implantation of highly loaded ^{125}I seeds [12].

The following is a report of our results after interstitial irradiation of brain metastases using ^{125}I seeds in a series of 20 patients.

Method

The procedure is carried out exclusively under stereotactic conditions. We use the Riechert-Mundinger* stereotactic system. The technique has been described elsewhere [2]. All operations were performed under local anaesthesia following mild sadation with diazepam (10 mg) and midazolam (2 mg). After the head ring had been positioned (Fig. 1), an enhanced (Jopamidol, 612 mg/kg body weight) CT scan was performed. The target point calculation was derived from the CT scans. Metastases are usually well visible in CT so that no stereotactic MRI scan was necessary. If the site of the lesion indicated the existence of a larger artery or heavy vascularization in the immediate vicinity, cerebral angiography was performed, also under stereotactic conditions. Biopsy was done in most cases from a frontal approach. A 5 × 5 cm-large area of skin was shaven and a local anaesthetic infiltrated. After incision of the skin a 3–8 mm burrhole was performed. A hollow cannula was advanced up to the target point. Using a special forceps several (3–9) 1 mm³-large samples were taken. Some of the samples were examined in May-Grünwald-Giemsa smear stain (Fig. 2) the others embedded in

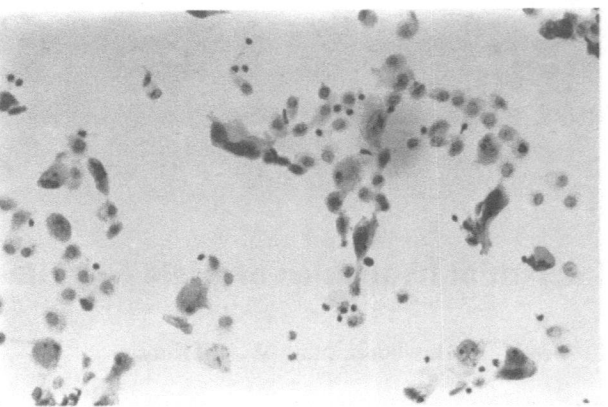

Fig. 2. Smear stain of a carcinoma of the lung (May-Grünwald-Giemsa staining). The diagnosis can be made on the basis of the intraoperative cytological examination. The remaining samples are stained and submitted to paraffin-histological investigation. Immunohistochemical tests are done if necessary

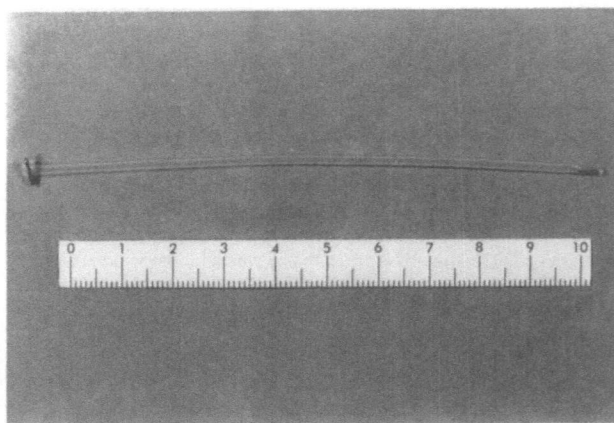

Fig. 3. The iodine seeds are sealed in a teflon catheter which shrinks under the application of heat. The catheter is removed after irradiation is completed

paraffin. Immunohistochemical tests were carried out when deemed necessary. Most of the metastases could already be identified in the cytological native test, so that the indication for interstitial radiotherapy could be made in the same session. The procedure for interstitial radiotherapy was as follows: a ^{125}I seed, from a special seed-bank harbouring multiple seeds with different activities, was sealed in the tip of a teflon catheter (Fig. 3) which shrinks after the application of heat and autoclaved at 134 °C, 2.5 bars for 40 minutes. The tip of the catheter was stereotactically positioned at the target point. The other end of the catheter was cut off at the level of the burrhole and secured with a small tantalum clip. The correct position of the seed was checked by X-ray performed under stereotactic conditions (Fig. 4). Afterwards, the incision was closed. In all cases the seeds were implanted temporarily and were removed after completion of radiotherapy. To remove the seed a 10 mm incision was performed under local anaesthesia and the catheter with the seed and tantalum clip were pulled out.

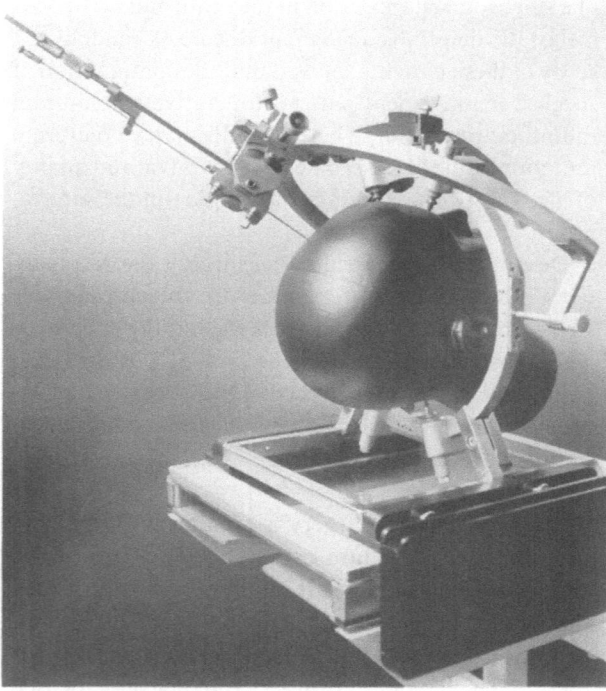

Fig. 1. Head ring of Riechert-Mundinger stereotactic system. The ring is secured to the patient's head with four posts under local anaesthesia

---

* Distributed by Leibinger GmbH, Freiburg, Germany.

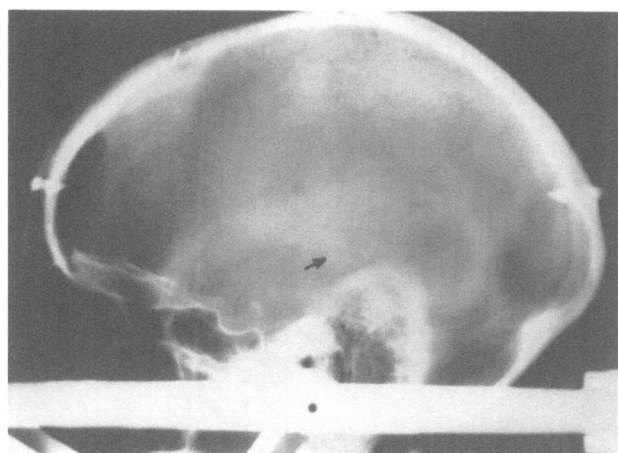

Fig. 4. ^{125}I seeds after implantation (arrow). The catheter is cut at the level of the burrhole and secured with a tantalum clip. The wound is then closed. For removal, the catheter along with the clip is subcutaneously located and pulled out

Table 2. *Location of the Metastasis (n = 20)*

Frontal	8
Parietal	5
Temporal	3
Central	1
Basal ganglia	2
Pontine	1

Table 3. *Site of the Primary Tumour (n = 19 Patients)*

Lung	8
Breast	3
Colon	3
Larynx	1
Renal	1
Thyroid gland	1
Occult	2

Patients and Material

A total of 20 interstitial implantations with ^{125}I seeds were carried out in 19 patients with cerebral metastases. The Karnofsky performance scores of the patients treated were between 60 and 90 percent (mean 80), the mean age was 54 years (range: 40–70) (Table 1). Eight metastases were frontal, five parietal, three temporal, one in the central region, and two in the area of the basal ganglia. One metastatic lesion was located in the pons (Table 2). The site of the primary tumour was the lung in eight cases (42%), the breast in three cases (16%), the colon in three cases (16%), the larynx in two cases (5%) (one patient had a second tumour after 8 month), the kidney in one case (5%), and the thyroid gland in one case (5%) (Table 3). In two cases (11%) the primary tumour was unknown. All of the metastases

Table 1. *Interstitial Irradiation of Brain Metastases: Characteristics*

	Median (range)
Karnofsky performance status (%)	80 (60–90)
Age (years)	54 (40–70)
Isotope	Iodine-125 (seed)[a]
Application	temporary
Tumour diameter (mm)	20 (14–24)
Activity (mCi)	8.8 (3.2–14.7)
Dose (cGy)	6000
Irradiation time (days)	28 (11–52)
Mean dose rate (cGy/h)	11 (5–22)

[a] Model 6702, Amersham International, Buckinghamshire, England

treated were spherical, which is a very conducive geometric form for interstitial radiotherapy. All of the lesions were irradiated with one single seed, which was positioned to the centre of the tumour. The tumour radius ranged from 14 to 24 mm (mean 20). The mean activity of the implanted ^{125}I seeds was 8.8 mCi (3.2–14.7) ($= 32,56*10^{10}$ Becquerel), the irradiated tumour diameter was 20 mm (14–24). The mean length of time the seeds remained indwelling was 28 days (11–52). The dose at the tumour margin in all patients was 6,000 cGy. The mean dose rate was 11 cGy/h (range: 5–22) (Table 1).

Results

The objective of radiosurgery is to necrotize and hence to devitalise the metastasis. The lesions were followed-up by CT scanning. The behaviour of the metastases varied considerably. In some cases there was a marked reduction in size (five cases) (Fig. 5), in other cases only a slight reduction (11 cases). In two patients the lesion size remained unchanged. One patient died during radiotherapy due to the primary tumour (lung) and therefore could not be examined by CT upon completion of the radiotherapy. At the time of his death, he had received only two-thirds of the 6000cGy originally planned. Histology of the brain showed a circumscribed central necrosis, surrounded by a concentric border of vital tumour cells (Fig. 6). The adjacent white matter showed moderate edema.

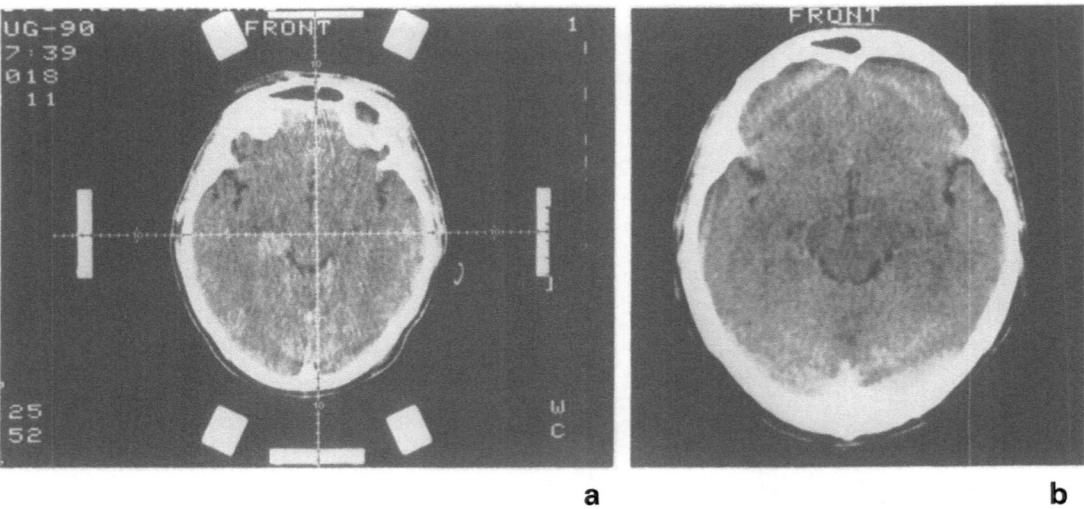

Fig. 5. (a) Metastasis of a carcinoma of the breast in the region of the left thalamus. (b) Complete remission after 40 days

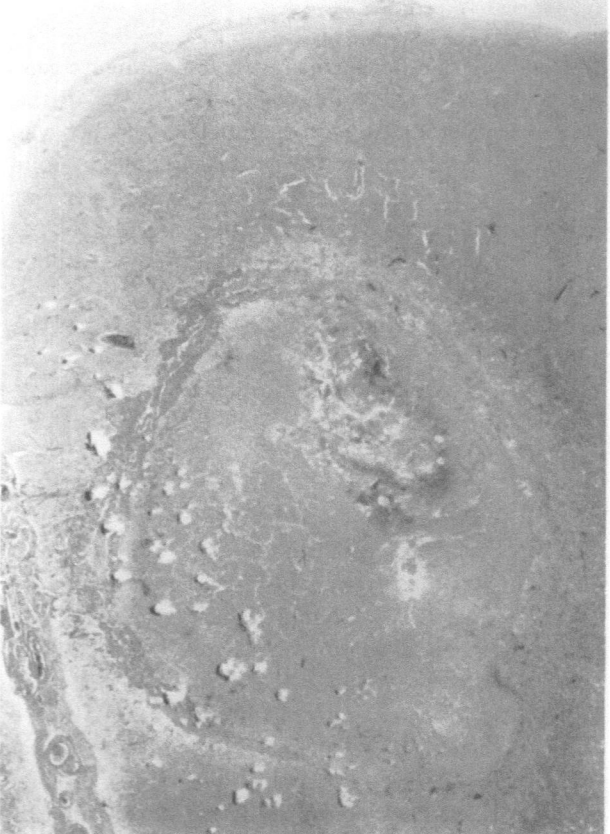

Fig. 6. Metastasis of a carcinoma of the lung. The patient died of non-neurologic causes before interstitial irradiation was completed. The histological examination shows a circumscribed central necrosis surrounded by a concentric border of vital tumour cells. The adjacent white matter shows moderate edema formation (elastica staining)

Table 4. *Advantages of Radiosurgical Treatment of Brain Metastases*

– Minimally invasive procedure
– Minimal damage to normal brain tissue
– No supplementary risk by anaesthesia
– No interference with other therapeutic modalities
– Low stress for the patient
– Short hospitalisation time (1–2 days)
– Low cost

Table 5. *Reasons Why Brain Metastases are Ideal for Interstitial Irradiation*

– They are often spherical
– Mostly relatively small (<3 cm) at presentation
– The normal brain parenchyma is displaced outside the potential radiosurgical target volume
– Minimally invasive growing

Since the stereotactic serial biopsy of the tumour had originally disclosed a solid, vital tumour, it can be assumed that these cells would also have become necrotic, had the irradiation been carried out to completion.

One patient developed a second metastasis on the contralateral side after having completed radiotherapy and having shown a good local response.

Only one patient in our series developed a local recurrence. The tumour grew along the track in which the teflon catheter with the ^{125}I seeds had been located. A review of the treatment protocol revealed that a very low dose rate had been chosen (6 cGy/h). No complications occurred, neither during biopsy, nor during the subsequent radiation therapy. Only one patient, who developed a metastasis in the central region, suffered a temporary worsening of an already existing hemiparesis, which was probably due to perifocal edema. The patient was given dexamethasone and the paresis improved. None of the patients died of neurologic causes.

Discussion

Interstitial radiotherapy is applied in neuro-oncology, especially to treat gliomas and is considered standard therapy [3, 11]. It is both an alternative as well as an adjuvant treatment to open surgical management. With interstitial radiotherapy a high local radiation dose can be delivered directly to the lesion while sparing the surrounding normal brain. When highly loaded seeds are applied, the method is also referred to as radiosurgery. The success in treating gliomas, as well as the minimal stress the stereotactic implantation of radioactive isotopes puts on the patient encouraged us to employ the method in patients with brain metastases. These lesions are usually circumscribed and spherical [8]. This makes them accessible to dosimetry. Metastases are frequently located in functionally critical areas of the brain, making them difficult to reach by open surgical resection. In addition, many patients are no candidates for general anaesthesia because of their general condition. The diagnosis of a single intracerebral lesion, which is suspected to be a metastasis can and must be confirmed by stereotactic biopsy in order to get a definitive histological diagnosis. The importance of a stereotactic biopsy, which has been stressed out by many authors [1, 7], was confirmed in our series by the following fact: Three patients, who were referred to us for interstitial irradiation of suspected brain metastases were not implanted because biopsy revealed that the lesions were not metastatic. One patient had an inflammatory process, the second a cerebral infarction, and the third patient a lymphoma. Lymphomas are not uncommon in patients with malignant disease because of their altered immune systems. The ability to obtain a histological diagnosis intraoperatively is an advantage of the method over radiosurgical convergent beam irradiation.

In the series presented we were able to treat brain metastases successfully with a method that puts little stress on the patient, however, it must be pointed out that this treatment is strictly palliative. The prognosis is dependent on the primary tumour. A randomised study showed that patients with solitary brain metastases treated with surgery plus whole-brain irradiation had a significantly longer survival than those treated with radiation alone. The goal of modern oncology, however, is not just to prolong survival, but also to maintain the quality of life. Radiosurgery has fewer risks in comparison with microsurgery and there is less strain put on the patient. The fact that the procedure can be carried out under local anaesthesia eliminates the problems concerning general anaesthesia in these patients, whose condition often makes them unable to undergo open surgery. Hospitalisation can be kept brief (usually not more than 2 to 3 days) and costs are far lower than with conventional surgery. Another advantage of the short postoperative hospitalisation period is that it allows the patients who are under current radio- or chemotherapy for their malignant disease to continue treatment according to schedule. Only one of the 20 patients in our series developed local progression. Subsequent microsurgical revision revealed that the irradiated volume was fully necrotic, but that the tumour had apparently continued to grow along the catheter track. The analysis of this case showed that a low dose rate (the lowest in this series) of 6 cGy/h and hence long irradiation period (45 days) had been chosen. Having learned from this, we now prefer to use a higher dose rate (>10 cGy/h) over a shorter irradiation period (<21 days).

Our series is too small to allow reliable conclusions to be made on the histology-specific behaviour of the size of the lesion under radiotherapy.

In our series only temporary seeds were employed. We consider these better than permanent implantation for several reasons: a more precise dosimetry can be achieved because the beginning and completion of irradiation can be exactly defined. The irradiation can be interrupted at any time, for example, if the seeds are not in the correct position, if side effects occur, or for reasons of radiation protection. In terms of radiation protection, the use of temporary implants is preferred since any restrictions apply only during the time of the irradiation. Due to the soft radiation from ^{125}I and the activities used in all patients the local dose rate at a distance of 1 meter was less than 1 μSv/h.

Because of our small number of patients, we cannot judge our results according to generally valid oncologic criteria. Nevertheless, the findings are promising and allow us to conclude that interstitial irradiation of brain metastases is an effective treatment which puts little strain on the patient and which does not interfere with other forms of therapy. It is an alternative to both open microsurgery as well as to radiosurgical convergent beam irradiation; not, however, to whole-brain irradiation.

Acknowledgements

The neuropathological evaluation was done by H. Budka, Neurological Institute, University of Vienna.

The autoptic material of Fig. 6 was evaluated by K. Rössler, Neurosurgical Department, University of Vienna.

References

1. Alesch F (1995) The role of stereotactic biopsy in radiosurgery. Acta Neurochir (Wien) [Suppl] 63: 20–24
2. Alesch F, Budka H, Kitz K, Koos W (1992) Die stereotaktische Biopsie von zerebralen Prozessen. Ergebnisse anhand einer Serie von 250 Fällen. Wien Klin Wochenschr 104: 67–72
3. Bernstein M, Gutin PH (1981) Interstitial irradiation of brain tumors: a review. Neurosurgery 9: 741–750
4. Cairncross JG, Kim JH, Posner JB (1980) Radiation therapy for brain metastases. Ann Neurol 7: 529–541
5. Cairncross JG, Posner JB (1983) The management of brain metastases. In: MD W (eds) Oncology of the nervous system. Martinus Nijhoff, Boston, pp 341–377
6. Coffey RJ, Flickinger JC, Bissonette DJ, Lunsford LD (1991) Radiosurgery for solitary brain metastases using the cobalt-60 gamma unit: methods and results in 24 patients. Int J Radiation Oncology 20: 1287–1295
7. Friedman WA, Sceats DJ, Nestok BR, Ballinger WE (1989) The incidence of unexpected pathological findings in an image-guided biopsy series: a review of 100 consecutive cases. Neurosurgery 25: 180–184
8. Loeffler JS, Alexander IE, Kooy HM, Wen PY, Fine HA, Black PM (1991) Radiosurgery for brain metastases. In: Principles and practice of oncology, Vol 5
9. Lunsford LD, Flickinger J, Linder G, Maitz A (1989) Stereo-tactic radiosurgery of the brain using the first united states 201 cobalt-60 source gamma knife. Neurosurgery 24: 151–159
10. Order SE, Hellman S, Von EC, Kligerman MM (1968) Improvement in quality of survival following whole-brain irradiation for brain metastasis. Radiology 91: 149–153
11. Ostertag C, Kreth FW (1992) Iodine-125 interstitial irradiation for cerebral gliomas. Acta Neurochir (Wien) 119: 53–61
12. Ostertag C, Weigel K, Warnke P, Lombeck G, Kleihues P (1983) Sequential morphological changes in the dog brain after interstitial iodine-125 irradiation, Neurosurgery 13: 523–528
13. Patchell RA, Tibbs PA, Walsh JW, Dempsey RJ, Maruyama Y, Kryscio RJ, Markesbery WR, MacDonald JS, Young B (1990) A randomized trial of surgery in the treatment of single metastases to the brain. Engl J Med 322: 494–500
14. Pickren J, Lopez G, Tsukada Y, Lane W (1983) Brain metastases: an autopsy study. Cancer Treat Symp 2: 295–313
15. Sauer R (1987) Radiation therapy of brain tumors. In: Jellinger K (eds) Therapy of malignant brain tumors. Springer, Wien New York, pp 195–276
16. Sause WT, Crowley JJ, Morantz R, Rotman M, Mowry PA, Bouzaglou A, Borst JR, Selin H (1990) Solitary brain metastasis: results of an RTOG/SWOG protocol evaluation surgery + RT versus RT alone. Am J Clin Oncol 13: 427–432
17. Sturm V, Kober B, Hover KH (1987) Stereotactic percutaneous single dose irradiation of brain metastases with a linear accelerator. Int J Radia Oncol Biol Phys 13: 279–282
18. Walker A, Robins M, Weinfeld F (1985) Epidemiology of brain tumors: the national survey of intracranial neoplasms. Neurology 35: 219–226
19. Zimm S, Wampler GL, Stablein D, Hazra T, Young HF (1981) Intracerebral metastases in solid-tumor patients. Natural history and results of treatment. Cancer 48: 384–394

Correspondence: François Alesch, M.D., Neurochirurgische Universitätsklinik, Währinger Gürtel 18–20, A-1090 Wien, Austria.

Acta Neurochir (1995) [Suppl] 63: 35–39

Optimization of Dose Distribution for LINAC Based Radiosurgery Using Elliptical Collimators

G. F. Popescu[1], **J. E. Rodgers**[1], and **R. von Hanwehr**[2]

[1]Department of Radiation Medicine, Georgetown University Medical Center and [2]Department of Neurosurgery, The Johns Hopkins University, Baltimore, ML, U.S.A.

Summary

The use of non-circular collimators is considered on all or some of the arcs used for radiosurgery on a linear accelerator in order to obtain conformal dose distribution for non-spherical lesions using a single isocenter. An extension of software to allow for use of non-circular collimators and a mathematical optimization based on prescribed doses on the lesion surface and on points in normal tissue (critical structures) are presented. Tests of the optimization method on simulated cases indicate that several boosts from selected positions along the arcs, superimposed on an optimized arc configuration allows one to obtain a highly conformal dose distribution with simple elliptical inserts. The optimization method can be applied to any type of collimation and is particularly effective with variable dose-rate machines.

Keywords: LINAC radiosurgery; dose distribution.

Introduction

Conventional Linear Accelerator (LINAC)-based neuroradiosurgery employs convergent noncoplanar arcs and circular collimators to generate highly focused, quasi-spherical dose distributions centered around a stereospatially-defined anatomical target point that is aligned coincident with the isocenter of the LINAC beam. In many clinical cases, anatomical lesion volumes have irregularly-shaped geometry, and irregular fields need to be shaped to conform to these irregular target lesion volumes. Although geoconformal dose distributions and protection of adjacent critical structures can be achieved to some extent by modifying arc and couch configuration, length, position and non-segmented arc dose weighting, these maneuvers may only significantly impact on the lower isodose level regions of a dose distribution. Alternatively, the use of

multiple overlapping targets is another approach that can result in a composite field with enhanced geoconformal dosimetry in the higher isodose regions. The inherent field overlap of the multiple target method can introduce dose inhomogeneities that may increase radiotoxicity [6].

The need to achieve geoconformal dosimetry without increasing dose volume inhomogeneity requires new approaches. Leavitt *et al.* [3] and McGinley *et al.* [4] presented a computer-controlled system of dynamically-adjustable, 4-jawed collimators for stereotactic radiosurgery, while other adjustable multi-leaf micro-collimator systems for multi-angle fixed point and shoot fractionated, stereotactic precision radiotherapy are also in use. Such dynamic or static field molding techniques can improve conformal dosimetry or may mitigate against dose inhomogeneity, but require a significant technical effort. Also Schlegel *et al.* [10] have presented a manual multileaf collimator which is adjusted for each arc based on a lesion projection solid model.

Suggested by Serago *et al.* [11] and, independently, by the present authors [8], an alternative approach is the use of non-circular collimation. However, the ability to accurately simulate elliptical fields and to evaluate the degree of geoconformal dosimetry and dose homogeneity achieved in tandem, requires appropriately compliant treatment planning software [13]. Accordingly, we present the extension of our radiosurgery treatment planning and virtual simulation system [12] to non-circular collimation, along with our model for concurrent mathematical optimization of geoconformal dose distribution for irregular lesions using a *single-target, non-circular collimation* approach. This optimization system is intended to identify and simulate preferred combinations of: 1) dose-weighted treatment arc segment configuration and 2) non-circular collimation parameters, that best correspond to a desired homogenous, geoconformal dose distribution.

Methods and Materials

1. Dose Computation for an Elliptical Collimator

Computation of dose to any point in the brain both represents a superposition of contributions from all arcs and is affected by the introduction of non-circular collimators. For circular cllimators, the point dose contribution, D, (arising from a gantry rotation arc segment, i.e. arc increment) may be calculated according to Rice *et al.* [9]:

$$D(d, s) = MS_t(c)[SAD/(SSD + d)]^2 TMR(d, \rho)R(s/\rho; c) \quad (1)$$

where:

d = geometric depth of the calculation point below the surface of a patient's scalp, along the central axis (CAX) of the beam,

s = radial distance perpendicular from CAX to a calculation point,

ρ = radial distance from CAX to the edge of the circular field projected at depth d,

R = off-axis ratio or beam profile for a collimator c,

M = monitor units delivered for the arc increment,

$S_t(c)$ = total scattering or output factor for the collimator c,

SAD = source axis distance,

SSD = source to skin distance along the CAX, and

TMR = tissue-maximum-ratio (for depth d and field size ρ).

It is assumed that the LINAC is calibrated to 1 cGy/MU at the depth of maximum dose, and that, in accordance with conventional algorithms for brain irradiations, tissue inhomogeneity corrections are not needed.

To extend the computation to non-circular collimators, the radial beam profile is replaced by a 2D-profile, $\mathcal{R}(r, \phi; c)$. The angle ϕ, defined in Fig. 1, subtends the projected collimator major axis with the direction from the CAX to the calculation point. Radial dose profiles were measured for a series of angles around the center of the ellipse, usually 30° apart, using film positioned at the isocenter. In order to obtain a profile, the dose point is projected along the beam line to the depth of the LINAC isocenter, and a linear interpolation between two adjacent table entries (positions) is used to estimate a profile falling between those two table positions. We have found it convenient to convert the film-derived digital optical density data to a 2D dose distribution by using an H&D curve and by then extracting twelve radial profiles from it. Precision-fashioned on a milling machine, our actual elliptical lead collimator insert has a rounded rectangular cross-section, rather than a true ellipse, and has a three stage taper for divergence.

In order to compute the dose contributions from arc increments (segments) to points inside the skull, the beam projection is translated to stereotactic frame coordinates. (The stereotactic coordinate system is defined by standard stereotactic frame axes: OZ – along the couch pointing to the cranial vertex; OX – pointing to the right with the patient supine; and OY anterior/posterior transecting the frame

origin). Next, we define, **V**, as the intersection of the gantry rotation plane with the beam's eye view-plane, II, shown in Fig 1. Thus, if the gantry axis is **G**, and the beam central axis is **P**, then the reference axis, **V**, is given by $\mathbf{V} = \mathbf{G} \times \mathbf{P}$. This choice leaves the axis **V** pointed to the left side of the head (see Fig. 2), provided the table is perpendicular to the gantry rotation plane. For the table at θ, **G** is calculated in stereotactic frame coordinates OX'Y'Z' by applying a rotation of the 'table' vector **Z** about a vertical axis **IY** which transects the isocenter. In the OX'Y'Z' stereotactic frame system we get $\mathbf{G} = (-\sin\theta, 0, \cos\theta)$. With P_1, P_2, and P_3 being the components of the "beam" vector, the reference axis is given by:

$$\mathbf{V} = \begin{vmatrix} \vec{i} & \vec{j} & \vec{k} \\ -\sin\theta & 0 & \cos\theta \\ P_1 & P_2 & P_3 \end{vmatrix}$$

$$= (-P_2\cos\theta, P_1\cos\theta + P_3\sin\theta, -P_2\sin\theta) \quad (2)$$

The program projects a dose point M along the X-ray source beam line and onto the beam's eye view plane that transects the target, computes the distance of the projection (M' in Fig. 1) to the target (coincident with the isocenter), and solves Eq. (2) for the angle Φ between IM' and **V**. The collimator orientation is given by the angle Ψ between **V** and the major axis of the ellipse (IA in Fig. 1).

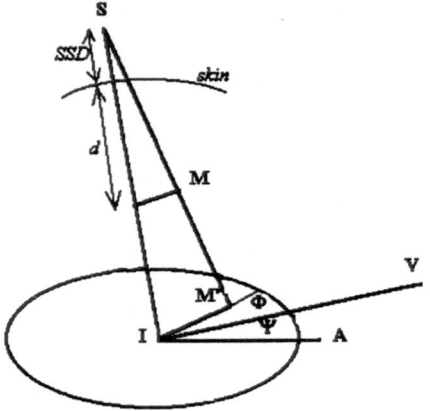

Fig. 1. Projection of a dose calculation point onto a beam's eye view plane through the isocenter

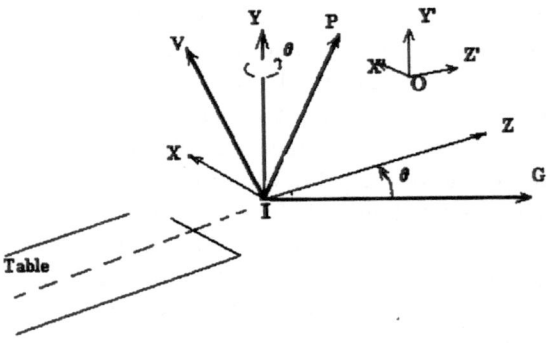

Fig. 2. Definition of reference axis **V**. The gantry rotation axis, **G**, and a beam direction, **P**, are drawn in the IXYZ system with the origin at the isocenter I. This system is parallel to the frame system OX'Y'Z'

Hence, the profile is selected by the angle $\phi = \Phi + \Psi$. Ψ is the extra degree of freedom gained by use of a non-circular collimator.

2. Optimization of Dose Distribution

Although the planning system extension used for methodological validation during this computer simulation supports use of a different circular or non-circular collimator for each arc, the optimization algorithm can support use of multiple collimators during different segments within an arc. Let us assume that a desired dose distribution, $\Delta(\mathbf{r}_i)$, $i = 1 \cdots N_L$ has been prescribed for the lesion, and that the prescribed dose limits to normal tissues, $\Delta(\mathbf{r}_j)$, $j = N_L + 1, \ldots N_L + N_C$, are specified for critical structures, including those close to the target. The total dose delivered to each such "prescription" point is a sum of the contributions from arc increments, as calculated by equation (1), with an extension supporting use of non-circular collimators:

$$D(\mathbf{r}) = \sum_{k=1}^{N_a} \sum_{i=\text{start}(k)}^{\text{end}(k)} w_{ki} D_{ki}(\mathbf{r}) \tag{3}$$

where: N_a is the number of arcs, and $D_{ki}(\mathbf{r})$ is the contribution of the i-th segment of the k-th arc to calculation point directed by $\mathbf{r}$.

We have assigned a weight, w_{ki}, representing the number of monitor units for the arc segment indexed by k and i, i.e. in a manner similar to the conformal therapy optimization approach proposed by Chung-Bin and Malyala [1]. If the gantry is in continuous motion, then a set of weights, $\{w_{ki}\}$, represents variable monitor unit dose rates for corresponding arc segments. We consider a dose distribution to be *optimal*, if it will minimize the discrepancies between the prescribed and computed doses to prescription points. In keeping with this approach, we have chosen:

$$F(\mathbf{w}) = \tfrac{1}{2}\alpha \sum_{i=1}^{N_L} f(\mathbf{w}; \overline{r}_i)^2 + \tfrac{1}{2}\beta \sum_{j=1}^{N_C} g(\mathbf{w}; \overline{r}_j)^2 \tag{4}$$

as the objective function to be minimized; the first sum denotes a lesion and the second denotes a critical structure; a sum of several terms may replace the second term in Eq. (4), when more than one critical structure is involved. α and β are user specified factors of "importance" indicating where the dose conformity is most desired. Since the residuals, $f(\mathbf{w}; \mathbf{r}_j)$ and $g(\mathbf{w}; \mathbf{r}_j)$, are linear functions of the unknown vector $\mathbf{w}$, we arrive at a linear least squares problem with constraints: $\mathbf{w}_k > = 0$. Following Weeks *et al.* [14], we define the residuals as follows:

$$f(\mathbf{w}; \overline{r}_i) = \begin{cases} D(\mathbf{w}; \overline{r}_i) - \Delta(\overline{r}_i), & D(\mathbf{w}; \overline{r}_i) > \Delta(\overline{r}_i) \\ 0, & D(\mathbf{w}; \overline{r}_i) \leqslant \Delta(\overline{r}_i) \end{cases} \tag{5a}$$

$$g(\mathbf{w}; \overline{r}_j) = \begin{cases} D(\mathbf{w}; \overline{r}_j) - \Delta(\overline{r}_j), & D(\mathbf{w}; \overline{r}_j) < \Delta(\overline{r}_j) \\ 0, & D(\mathbf{w}; \overline{r}_j) \geqslant \Delta(\overline{r}_j) \end{cases} \tag{5b}$$

With some algebraic manipulation, Eq. (4) may be reformulated, up to a constant term irrelevant for solving the minimization problem, as:

$$F_1(\overline{w}) = \tfrac{1}{2}\overline{w}^T \cdot G \cdot \overline{w} + \overline{C}^T \cdot \overline{w} \tag{6}$$

where the elements of the symmetric matrix G are defined as:

$$G_{lm} = \alpha \sum_{i=1}^{N_L} D_{li} \cdot D_{mi} + \beta \sum_{j=1}^{N_C} D_{lj} \cdot D_{mj} \tag{6a}$$

and where the elements of the vector $\mathbf{C}$ are defined as follows:

$$C_m = -\alpha \sum_{i=1}^{N_L} D_{mi} \cdot \Delta(\overline{r}_i) - \beta \sum_{j=1}^{N_C} D_{mj} \cdot \Delta(\overline{r}_j) \tag{6b}$$

Eq. (6) is essentially a multivariable quadratic objective function. "Reasonable" upper bounds on optimization variables complete the constraints.

3. Optimization Software and Strategy

Despite the relatively large number of variables (around 100) in our problem, recent progress in research for solutions of quadratic programming problems (q.v., the monograph of Moré and Wright [6]) has made it possible to tackle this type of problem. We have used an efficient code for large-scale problems, the program 'BQPD'. It is based on a study of Fletcher and implements active set methods [2].

We have devised a simple strategy for arc selection with elliptical collimators: The target, I, is set at the lesions's center-of-gravity. Let AB be the maximum chord defined by the lesion surface: a plane, Γ, that passes through I while perpendicular to AB, defines the "principal" arc; the major axis of the ellipse is perpendicular to the gantry rotation plane for this arc. A plane, Ω, perpendicular to Γ, through I, defines the second arc; the minor axis of the ellipse is perpendicular to the latter plane for this arc. The procedure determines optimized arc segment delimiters and their dose weights $\{w_{ki}\}$, as well as optimum couch positions around the bisectors of those angles made by the planes and Ω. Usually, the determination of couch positions presents a combinatorial optimization problem. Our approach calculates the objective function $F_1(\mathbf{w})$ and the corresponding arc segment dose weights $\{w_{ki}\}$ for couch position pairs in a range of angles around the above bisectors at 5° intervals.

To examine the various aspects of such a complex problem, our computer software simulated CT-cuts for an ellipsoid-shaped head containing lesions with irregular volume geometry. Lesions were positioned at various intracranial locations and orientations. Using vector-based dose calculation points overlaid on rasterized anatomical imagery, the 3D surface of the lesion volume, an appropriate stereotactic target point, and the desired dose coverage were all defined. A set of maximal dose tolerance calculation points, representing a critical structure that would be relevant to the lesion's position in a real-world anatomical context, were similarly defined. Prescribed lesion surface dose was 10 Gy and the tolerance dose on "critical points" adjacent to the lesion was 2 Gy. Cued by target-centered orthogonal beam's-eye-view and beam perspective projections of lesion and critical structure cross-section, collimator shapes and diameters were iteratively selected. The simulation was now optimized to determine 'best': arc stop/start delimiters, arc segment dose weights $\{w_{ki}\}$ in monitor units/degree, couch positions i.e. arc positions (as described above), and collimator orientation for gantry arcs *not* in Γ or Ω planes for each arc. [i.e. by optimizing for each orientation and by taking the minimum value of the objective function $F_1(\mathbf{w})$ into account].

4. Summary of Results and Observations

In designing validation cases for this algorithm, we observed two underlying objectives: the simplicity of the simulated treatment plan, and its applicability to various LINAC dose delivery control features. Accordingly, our model is constructed to achieve flexible arc segment dose delivery by superimposing optimized arc segment dose boosts over a continuously-dosed, underlying set of four convergent arcs. For the purposes of this study, we chose not to exceed four arcs, and we restricted simulation to one circular or non-circular (elliptical) collimator size and shape, and one collimator axis orientation per arc. The algorithm is, nevertheless, capable of handling dynamic, computer controlled variation of non-circular collimator axis orientation as well as many more arcs (subsequently retaining only a few in

Table 1. *Results for Five Optimization Cases, Rows A–E.* Columns 5–6 show the difference between calculated and prescribed dose averaged on prescription points on the lesion and critical structure, respectively. Columns 7–8 give the maximum absolute difference as percentage of the respective prescribed dose

Case	Lower bound	Objective funct. F	Boosts (#)	Dose av. dev. Lesion	Cr. st.	Dose max. dev. Lesion	Cr. str.
A	0	11,000	22	0.013%	—	0.399%	—
B	15	68,300	5	0.22%	—	9.515%	—
C	13	33,500	4	0.123%	—	7.086%	—
D	0	17,900	20	0.054%	0.712%	0.485%	6.035%
E	10	51,400	6	0.261%	0	5.156%	0

decreasing order of the average weight per arc or in order of decreasing major regional dose contributions by specific, individual arc segments).

Table 1 summarizes simulated optimization results. Each row (labelled "cases" A–E) represents an optimization. Initially, in case A, we imposed 0 as the lower bound condition for all arc segment dose weights, thus yielding 22 out of 96 arc segments with non-zero weights – a configuration providing a quasi-perfect conformal dose distribution. However, this generated a 'skipping' point and shoot arc segment dosing pattern that would require variable dose capabilities in a moving arc i.e., replacing the desired model of convergent, continuous dose rate, intersecting arcs. In order to maintain the convergent dynamic arc technique we proceeded to select a higher value than 0 for the lower bound in cases B and C, and the solution of the optimization problem now yielded the desired model. Specifically, only a few arc segments with monitor unit/degree weights greater (in fact, significantly greater) than the imposed lower bound emerged. These represent dose boosts delivered to optimized segments of the four underlying arcs whose already constant dose rate is equivalent to the imposed non-negative (> 0) lower bound. With Case C, only four optimized "boosts" to segments of four arcs are required to feasibly deliver a highly conformal and homogenous dose distribution. A similar trend was noted for the simulations D and E which included constraints on a critical organ close (about 1 cm) to the lesion. One should note that, since the problem is convex, the optimization procedure yields a *global minimum*. This minimum is smaller for cases A and D. In case E, even though all doses on the critical structure turned out to be smaller than the prescribed limit, the overall distribution is closer to the prescribed one.

Discussion

Although the non-circular, single-target features of our technique provide a high-degree of dose homogeneity in all five simulation case types, (A–E above), the approach of cases A and D yielded the best conformity. However, implementation would require impractical fixed arc segment techniques on conventional LINAC's, or systems providing dynamic variable dose delivery or 'skip and shoot' capability during execution of an arc. Thus, cases C and E are more desirable and achievable with present state-of-the-art LINAC systems.

Non-circular collimation techniques present distinct advantages for non-spherical lesions. They introduce an extra degree of freedom that facilitates optimization of geoconformal dose distribution with minimal dose inhomogeneity and without use of multiple isocenters. Also we have demonstrated that an arc segment weighting scheme using elliptical collimators provides flexibility in protecting critical structures. This flexibility includes switching between circular and non-circular collimators for various arcs or even arc segments. Beam's-eye-view graphic displays can aide during computer simulation with the selection of collimator shape.

This approach has some minor disadvantages. A repertoire of non-circular collimator shapes and sizes is required to achieve a fully versatile implementation of this approach. As well their use requires care be taken to properly account for the extra degree of freedom, the collimator angle, at all times.

Finally, an advantage of this approach is a mathematical optimization replacing the conventional trial and error approach. Starting with a desired, conformal dose distribution this *single-target, non-circular collimation* model provides an extension of the earlier simulation software to include support for both elliptical collimators and for concurrent mathematical optimization of arc segment configuration and arc segment dose weighting parameters.

Acknowledgements

The authors thank Prof. R. Fletcher (Univ. of Dundee, UK) for making available his program BQPD and Dr. K. Weeks (Duke Univ. SC) for an extended abstract of his work [14].

References

1. Chung-Bin A, Malyala R (1987) Optimization of conformation-therapy by variation of dose rate. In: Bruinvis, Van Der Giessen, Van Klefens Wittkämper (eds) The use of computers in radiation therapy. North-Holland, pp 223–226

2. Fletcher R (1991) Resolving degeneracy in quadratic programming. Numerical analysis report NA/135, Department of Mathematics and Computer Science, University of Dundee, Dundee, Scotland, UK

3. Leavitt DD, Gibbs Jr FA, Heilburn MP, Moeller, JH and Takach GA (1991) Dynamic field shaping to optimize stereotactic radiosurgery. Int J Radiat Oncol Biol Phys 21: 1247–1255

4. McGinley PH, Butker EK, Crocker IR and Aiken R (1992) An adjustable collimator for stereotactic radiosurgery. Phys Med Biol 37: 413–419

5. Moré JJ, Wright SJ (1993) Optimization Software Guide, SIAM, Philadelphia

6. Nedzi LA, Kooy H, Alexander E, Loeffler JS (1990) Variables associated with the development of complications from radiosurgery of intracranial tumors (Abstr.). Int J Radiat Oncol Biol Phys 19: 249

7. Pike GB, Podgorsak EB, Peters TM, Pla C, Olivier A, Souhami L (1990) Dose distribution in radiosurgery. Med Phys 17: 296–304

8. Popescu GF, Rodgers JE, von Hanwehr, R (1991) Dose distribution by non-circular collimators for radiosurgery with a linear accelerator (Abstr.) Med Phys 18: 848

9. Rice RK, Hansen JL, Svensson GK, Siddon RL (1987) Measurement of dose distributions in small beams of 6 MV x-rays. Phys Med Biol 32: 1087–1099

10. Schlegel W, Pastyr O, Bortfeld T, Becker G, Schad L, Gademann G, and Lorenz WJ (1992) Computer systems and mechanical tools for stereotactically guided conformation therapy with linear accelerators, Int J Radiat Oncol Biol Phys 24: 781–787

11. Serago CF, Lewin AA, Houdek PV, Gonzales-Arias S, Abitbol AA, Marcial-Vega VA, Pisciotti V, Schwade JG (1991) Improved linac distributions for radiosurgery with elliptically shaped fields. Med Phys 21: 1321–1325

12. von Hanwehr R, Popescu GF, Rodgers JE (1994) Virtual simulator development for optimized radiosurgery. In: Pernecksky A (ed) Proc 1st Int Congress on Minimal Invasive Techniques in Neurosurgery, Wiesbaden, Germany June 15–10, 1993 (Abstr.). MITIN (1), Thieme

13. van Hanwehr R (1991) Frontiers of graphics supercomputer technology and advanced visualization guidance simulation software development for LINAC radiosurgery. In: Steiner (ed) Radiosurgery – Baseline and Trends, Raven, pp 25–47

14. Weeks KJ, Marks L, Ray SK, Spencer DP, Turner DA and Friedman AH (1991) 3D optimization of multiple arcs for stereotactic radiosurgery (Abstr.). Med Phys 18: 602

Correspondence: George F. Popescu, Ph.D., Department of Radiation Therapy, Georgetown University Medical Center, 3800 Reservoir Road, NW, Washington DC 2007–2197, U.S.A.

Acta Neurochir (1995) [Suppl] 63: 40–43

A Prototype Device for Linear Accelerator-Based Extracranial Radiosurgery

A. J. Hamilton[1,2] and **B. A. Lulu**[2]

[1] Section of Neurosurgery, Department of Surgery and [2] Department of Radiation Oncology,
University of Arizona Health Sciences, Tucson, AZ, U.S.A.

Summary

A prototype frame for accurate stereotactic localization and linear accelerator (LINAC)-based treatment of extracranial targets was developed. The ECRSF is designed to employ either spinal or skeletal osseous fixation to immobilize the area of interest and then encircle the targeted region with a traditional orthogonal, three-axis system. A series of experiments (n = 5) with semi-radiolucent calibration targets (n = 15) and computed tomography (CT) scanning using the EC showed that a mean localization error of $0.98 +/- 0.22$ mm was obtainable in the last two and most accurate series of experiments with these targets (n = 8). Using the LINAC to irradiate these same targets demonstrated an overall radiation treatment accuracy ranging from 1.4 to 2.0 mm. This discrepancy between localization error and overall radiation treatment error can be explained by a lack of isocentricity of the LINAC treatment which is typically less than 1 mm and can be as low as 0.5 mm. These data demonstrate that extracranial stereotactic radiosurgery is now technically feasible and that the accuracy of such treatment would be acceptable for clinical treatment.

Keywords: Extracranial stereotaxis; LINAC; radiosurgery; spinal stereotaxis; stereotaxis; stereotactic frame.

Introduction

While the applications for cranial radiosurgery have flourished since the first intracranial radiosurgery was first introduced by Lars Leksell in 1951 [2, 3], extracranial applications of existing hardware have been restricted to caudad extensions of cranially-fixed hardware [1]. We report a prototype design, an extracranial stereotactic radiosurgical frame (ECSRF), which permits extracranial stereotactic irradiation and employs skeletal fixation outside of the cranium. A series of experiments was undertaken to determine the accuracy of radiographic localization and radiosurgical treatment with this prototype ECSRF.

The objectives for the prototype design were:

(1) The accuracy of the system had to approximate or equal that which was already in clinical use for cranial systems.

(2) In order to achieve such accuracy, the system would require skeletal fixation rather than be a so-called 'frameless' or 'non-invasive' technology.

(3) The system must permit stereotactic irradiation of any target outside of the cranium.

(4) The system must be compatible with existing computed tomography (CT) and linear accelerator (LINAC) hardware in current clinical radiosurgical use.

(5) The device had to be capable of being employed for human use.

Description of Device

The device encloses the patient. It employs a rigid box 50 cm wide, 200 cm long and 18 cm deep which can be accommodated within an enclosing CT scanner bore of 56 cm in diameter (see Fig. 1). The x-y plane (i.e. that of a transverse or axial CT slice) is determined by the plane of the CT scanner field guide light. The x-z plane (i.e. that of a coronal slice) is fixed by leveling the rigid box in both the right-left axis and the cephalad-caudad axis with a high precision ($+/-1/1000$ of an inch over six inches) machinist's level. These two reference planes establish an orthogonal coordinate system. The origin of this coordinate system is defined as the center of a 12 mm plastic calibration sphere placed as closely as possible to the intended treatment target.

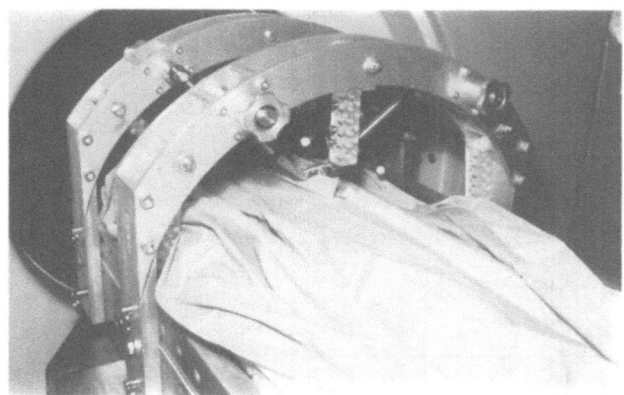

Fig. 1. The ECSRF inside the bore of CT scanner

to assure proper alignment of the x-y plane as determined by CT with the plane of LINAC gantry rotation (see Fig. 3). The LINAC table is then translated in three axes so that the guide lasers are aligned on the calibration target employed as the origin. This process completes the transfer of coordinates from CT to treatment machine. The coordinates of actual targets (real or phantom) is derived by software from the CT images as offsets in the x, y and z axes from the arbitrarily positioned calibration target designated as the origin. The LINAC treatment is again translated by these

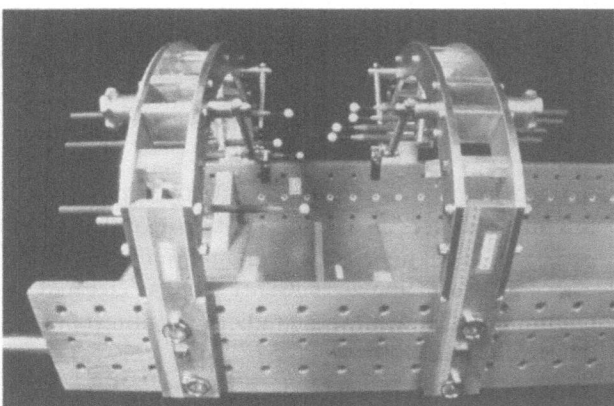

Fig. 2. Lateral view of the ECSRF with metal arches affixed and bolted to sides of the device. Holes show the range over which the arches may be moved to accommodate variable location along the axis of the body

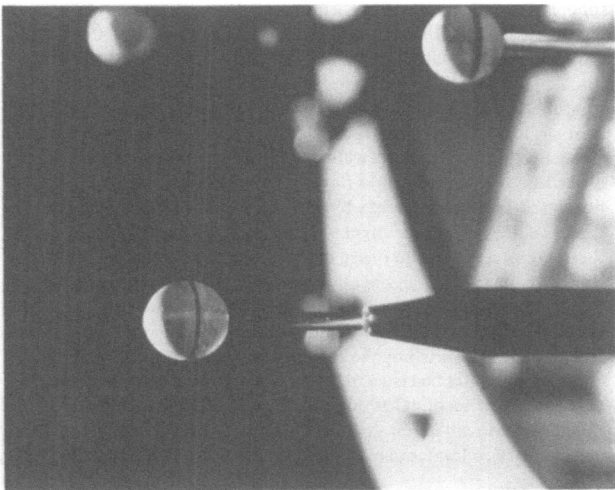

Fig. 3. Projection of orthogonal laser sighting system employed to align ECSRF for LINAC treatment (see text)

The scale factor for CT-derived magnification is obtained by direct film measurement and is also independently verified by measuring an object of known dimensions which is embedded within the frame.

The ECSRF employs two semi-circular metal arches which can be rigidly secured anywhere along the length of the device (see Fig. 3). The radiosurgical target is immobilized by skeletal fixation above and below the region of interest. This immobilization can be achieved either by means of osseous screws or by a prototype clamp which secures transcutaneously to the spinous process (see Fig. 4).

Once the coordinates for a designated target have been derived from CT scan images, the ECSRF is then transferred to a LINAC treatment table and leveled in x-z plane. The LINAC orthogonal guide lasers are used

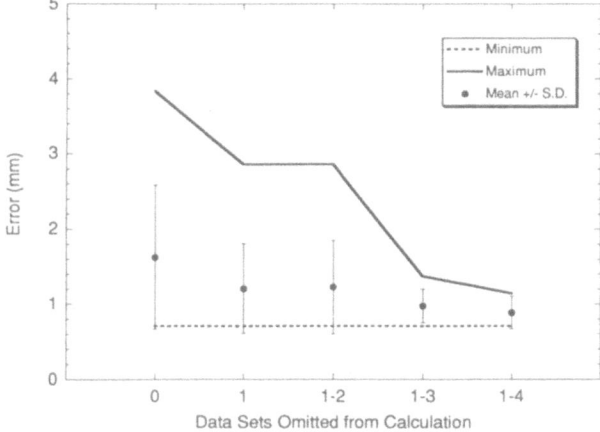

Fig. 4. Localization error. Mean, standard deviation, minimum and maximum values for CT-based localization error in millimeters as a function of the number of data sets that were used from successive experimental runs (see text)

calculated offsets so as to bring the designated target to isocenter (treatment position).

Methods

To test the accuracy of the ECSRF for both CT-derived localization of targets as well as LINAC treatment, a series of five independent experiments was carried out with a total of 15 spherical (12 mm diameter) radiolucent phantom targets. The targets were mounted randomly within the space between the two metal fixation arches. A single calibration target was then chosen as the designated coordinate origin. The ECSRF was placed and aligned in the CT scanner (Siemens Somatome) and the entire volume of interest between the metal archways was scanned every 2 mm in 2 mm thick slices. The x, y and z offsets relative to the designated origin for the phantom spheres were then determined from the CT images.

The ECSRF was then placed and aligned on the LINAC treatment table (Varian Clinac 6/100, Palo Alto, CA). The table was then translated in the x, y and z axes so as to align the orthogonal laser sighting system on the designated origin. For each phantom target in turn, the LINAC treatment table was translated to the coordinates as calculated from CT. If there were no measurement errors in the entire procedure then there would have been perfect correspondence between the position achieved by the guide lasers and the geometric center of the phantom target spheres. The localization error was therefore derived as the offset of the orthogonal cross hairs established by the sighting lasers and the center of the phantom spheres.

Total treatment error must also account for lack of perfect correspondence between the center of the radiation beam and the isocenter point as designated by the orthogonal guide lasers. Therefore, an additional error called isocentricity error was factored into accuracy calculations to account for this discrepancy. This error was added to our derived localization error both linearly and in quadrature to arrive at two estimates of overall treatment accuracy for the ECSRF.

Results

A. Localization Error

The results of the series of five experimental runs are summarized in Fig. 4 which depicts the mean and standard deviation values in CT-based localization error in millimeters plotted against the number of data sets that were used in the calculations. There was a decrease in localization error over the course of the series. Omitting the three earliest data sets and employing the final and most accurate experiments, a mean CT-derived localization error of 0.98 $=/-0.22$ mm was achieved for eight different targets. Combining the data from all five series yielded a mean localization error of 1.6 mm $+/-0.96$ mm.

B. Total Radiation Treatment Error

The data for total radiation treatment error are depicted in Fig. 5. For a given localization error of

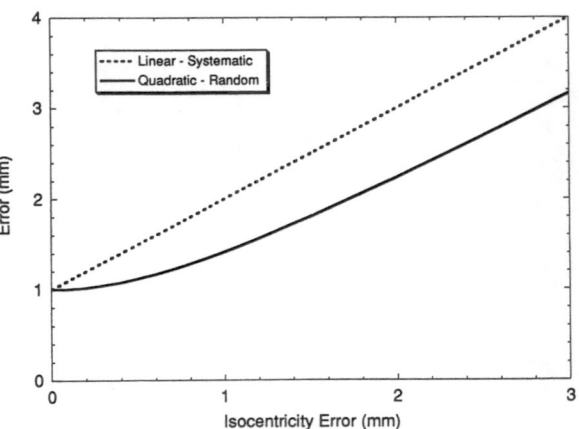

Fig. 5. Total treatment error (localization error = 1.0 mm). Overall LINAC-based radiation treatment error in millimeters as a function of isocentricity error for a given localization error of 1.00 mm using both a linear and quadratic model for factoring in isocentricity error (see text)

1.00 mm (see above) and an isocentricity error factored in a linear fashion, an overall radiation treatment error of 2.0 mm is obtained. This would represent the worst case scenario. If the isocentricity error is factored in quadrature, then the overall radiation treatment error falls to 1.4 mm as shown.

Discussion

This study shows that the prototype ECSRF has a total treatment accuracy comparable to that achieved with LINAC for intracranial applications [4].

The mean localization improved dramatically from the first through the third experimental runs. This was achieved by improving laser alignment and by properly accounting for CT and LINAC table 'sag' in both longitudinal and lateral planes. It was also found that the calibration sphere employed as the designated origin should be as close as possible to the intended treatment target to reduce errors produced by translation incurred by the LINAC table. Commercially available LINAC treatment tables with CT-scanner quality translation accuracy would also further reduce our localization error.

Isocentricity errors are machine-dependent and can be as low as 0.5–1.00 mm for new and well-adjusted equipment [4]. Conservative estimates of our own LINAC equipment yielded an isocentricity error nearly 3 times larger than what can be currently achieved. Isocentricity error was factored linearly and in quadrature to give the most reasonable range of treatment error. If the isocenter error is strictly correlated with the localization error then the errors must be added together in a linear fashion. If, on the other hand, the isocentricity error is independent of localization error (as would be the case if the treatment isocenter wandered about the nominal isocenter as the gantry and table rotate during treatment) then the errors can be added in quadrature.

These data lead us to conclude that extracranial stereotactic radiosurgery is technically feasible and that the overall treatment accuracy would range between 1.4 mm in the best case scenario and 2.0 mm in the worst case scenario with this prototype extracranial stereotactic frame. This level of treatment accuracy is accurate enough for most clinical application. Further studies are underway to document the ability of the frame to achieve adequate skeletal stabilization to permit clinical use.

Acknowledgments

Dr. Hamilton is a recipient of a Clinical Oncology Career Development Award from the American Cancer Society.

References

1. Hitchcock E (1969) An apparatus for stereotactic spinal surgery. Lancet 1:705–706
2. Leksell L (1951) The stereotaxic method and radiosurgery of the brain. Acta Chir Scand 102:316–319
3. Leksell L (1971) Stereotaxis and radiosurgery – an operative system. Thomas, Springfield
4. Luxton G, Petrovich Z, Jozsef G, Nedzi LA, Apuzzo MLJ (1993) Stereotactic radiosurgery: principles and comparison of treatment methods. Neurosurgery 32:241–259

Correspondence: Allan J. Hamilton, M.D., Department of Surgery, University of Arizona Health Sciences Center, Room 4411, 1501 N. Campbell Ave., Tucson, AZ, 85724, U.S.A.

Acta Neurochir (1995) [Suppl] 63: 44–51

Stereotactic Convergent Beam Radiosurgery Versus Stereotactic Conformation Beam Radiotherapy

G. Becker[1], W. Schlegel[2], J. Major[3], E. H. Grote[4], and M. Bamberg[1]

[1]Radiotherapy Department, University of Tübingen, [2]German Cancer Research Center, Heidelberg, [3]Department of Medical Physics, University of Tübingen, and [4]Neurosurgery Department, University of Tübingen, Federal Republic of Germany

Summary

By means of preliminary results in the treatment of patients with acoustic neurinoma the achievable accuracies, dose distributions and time consumption of stereotactic LINAC-based convergent beam radiosurgery are compared to those achieved with fractionated stereotactic conformation beam radiotherapy. Characteristics of both techniques are described. With the Tübingen radiosurgery system a good adaptation of the dose distribution to spherical or oval target volumes with a steep dose gradient was achieved, whereas homogeneity and adaptation of the dose distribution to irregularly shaped targets were better with the Heidelberg conformation technique. The mechanical accuracy of the Tübingen floorstand system was 0.3 mm +/− 0.2 mm, and that of the Heidelberg mask fixation system < 1 mm. Both methods require similar total treatment times. Nine patients were treated by the Tübingen radiosurgery system. The results are compared with 12 patients treated by conformation radiotherapy in Heidelberg. In both patient groups no further tumour growth occurred. Four of 9 single dose treated patients developed side-effects, such as temporary trigeminal and facial paraesthesia hearing deterioration and oedema. In contrast, patients treated by fractionated radiotherapy showed no side-effects.

Relating to the short follow-up the results indicate that single dose application has certain drawbacks for special indications. Further studies have to work out which method gives the best treatment results.

Keywords: Stereotaxy; radiosurgery; conformation radiotherapy.

I. Introduction

Stereotactic radiosurgery techniques, like GAMMA-Knife radiosurgery developed in 1951 by Leksell and the linear accelerator-based convergent beam irradiation technique developed in the last 10 years by different groups [2, 8, 12, 20, 23, 30], have become wide spread and successfull clinical methods [1]. At the University Hospital in Tübingen a convergent beam technique based on the radiosurgery system developed at the University of Florida in Gainesville [17] has been applied since 1991, particularly for patients with solitary brain metastasis, AVM and acoustic neurinoma. However, radiosurgical methods have also clear limitations. Irradiation with circular fields result in spherical or oval dose distributions. Adaptation of the dose to irregular shaped target volumes, like convex-concave shaped large acoustic neurinomas with intrameatal parts, metastases, meningiomas or large AVMs can be performed by treatment with several isocenters, but this will cause dose inhomogeneities. Furthermore, classical radiosurgery means a single dose application and is therefore limited to small volumes. Only AVMs seem to respond better to a high single dose than to fractionated radiotherapy [14, 15, 21, 26, 36]. However, it is not yet clear if this applies to other tumours as well. These drawbacks of radiosurgery have led to the development of the stereotactically guided fractionated conformation radiotherapy in the German Cancer Research Center (DKFZ) in Heidelberg. The technique is based on the stereotactic convergent beam irradiation and has been applied in Heidelberg since the late 1988. Fractionation is achieved by using a mask fixation system. Conform dose distributions are obtained with a multi-leaf-collimator and non-coplanar beams [32].

In this work the Tübingen convergent beam radiosurgery is compared to the Heidelberg conformation technique. By means of preliminary results in the treatment of patients with acoustic neurinoma, the achievable accuracies, dose distributions and time consumptions of both techniques are demonstrated and evaluated.

II. Material and Methods

1. *Stereotactic Convergent Beam Radiosurgery*

Stereotactic convergent beam radiosurgery in Tübingen is performed with the SRS 200-system (Philips), an independent sub system (Fig. 1), which can be attached to any linear accelerator type. The radiosurgical system is a modification of the Gainesville-system, which is described in detail elsewhere [17]. Hardware components of the SRS 200 are listed in Table 1.

Fixation system: Similar to classical radiosurgery the patient is fixed with screws drilled into the skull for perfect immobilization. A floorstand connecting patient, gantry and accelerator head is used, in order to attain a high precision of treatment delivery and stringent control of inherent positional inaccuracies of the radiation beam and the patient's position.

Localization components are based on the Brown-Robert-Wells (BRW)-Stereotactic-System modified by Cosman. Standard parts such as head frame, angiographic and CT localizer, which were improved in their mechanical accuracy, are applied in the usual fashion.

Virtual treatment planning is performed on efficient computers with three-dimensional dose representation.

Table 1. *Hardware Used for Stereotactic Convergent Beam Radiotherapy*

Mechanics	—SRS 200, Philips
	—based on BRW-stereotactic system
	—applied on a linear accelerator Philips SL 25
Hardware	—SUN 32 bit workstation
	—24 Mbyte ram
	—688 Mbyte disk
	—Array processor 4 Mbyte ram
	—colour monitor
	—1/2" tape streamer
	—1/4" Cartridge tape drive
Periphery	—digitizer
	—colour copier
	—laser printer
Imaging	—CT Siemens somatom DRH
	—MR Siemens magnetom 1, 5 T
	—Angio Siemens angioskop D

The target volume is defined in the central beam CT-slice and in sagittal reconstructions.

Dose calculation includes a pencil beam algorithm. Thus, the geometrical calculation base represents a 3-dimensional (3D) model, but the dose distributions are only calculated 2-dimensionally (2D), without correction of inhomogeneity and consideration of scattered radiation.

Presentation and evaluation of dose distribution: The isodose distribution can be overlayed to any axial CT slice, each arcing plane and frontal and sagittal isocenter reconstruction either as isodose lines or colour-washed areas. For the quantitative presentation a 2D dose profile is available, which represents a percentage dose profile at any point.

The transfer of the stereotactic target point coordinates to the patient is checked by a stereotactical fine-needle-system using the "target ball method" described by Lutz *et al.* [25].

Convergent beam radiosurgery: Concentration of the dose in the target volume is achieved by several non-coplanar moving beam techniques (arcs). Precision of the collimator motion during gantry and table movement is controlled by two bearings, one for the isocentric accuracy of the collimator, the other for the rotation of the head of the BRW-floorstand. The subsystem itself defines the mechanical treatment accuracy, since the beam collimator is not rigidly coupled to the radiation head of the LINAC. A gimble-type bearing with a sliding collimator mount is used to avoid any torque transfer from the LINAC head.

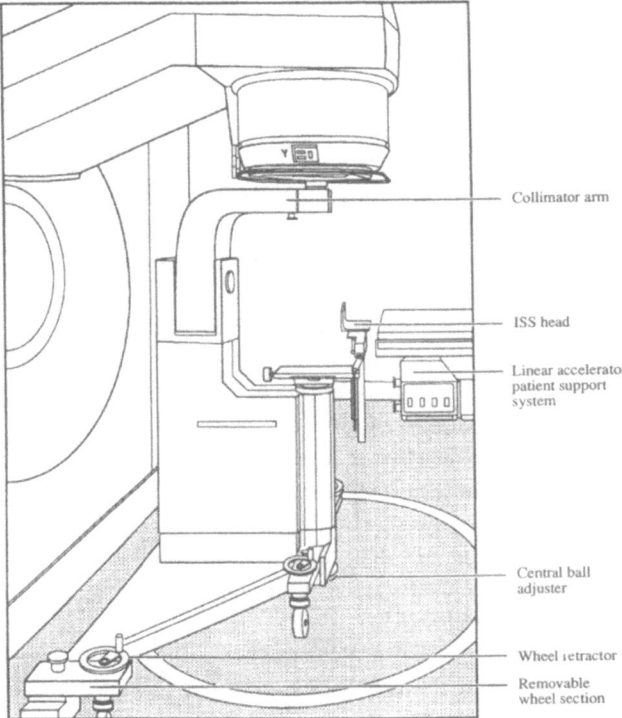

Collimator arm

ISS head

Linear accelerator patient support system

Central ball adjuster

Wheel retractor

Removable wheel section

Fig. 1. Isocentric sub-system

After determining a preliminary isocenter, the irradiation arcs can be selected within the movement limits defined by the sub-system. In Tübingen 7 arcs for one isocenter and a spherical target volume considering the limits of possible gantry and table movements are delivered (Table 2).

Quality assurance: During each application and treatment procedure a detailed analysis of the treatment accuracy including planning and dose delivery is performed. For test measurements a special head phantom was developed consisting of two plexiglass hemispheres and a set of test discs, which can be placed in between. In this way dosimetry by film, thermoluminescence or ionization chamber can be carried out without changing the geometry of the phantom set up.

2. Stereotactic Conformation Beam Radiotherapy

The limitations of radiosurgery and radiobiological problems of single dose application led to the development of computer systems and mechanical tools for stereotactically guided conformation therapy at the DKFZ, which are described in detail in [32, 33]. Hardware components are listed in Table 3.

Fixation system: An individually formed, removable and relocatable mask consisting of self-hardening plastic bandages of cast material (e.f. Scotch-Flex) immobilizes the patients' head and neck during the imaging procedure and the daily irradiations. The bandages fit closely to the head of the patient and are attached to the stereotactic base frame by wooden brackets [19, 32].

The localization system is based on the Riechert-Mundinger-frame, which has been modified for stereotactic irradiations [37]. The localization unit consists of plexiglass squares with integrated markers, which serve as landmarks for the stereotactic co-ordinate system [29].

Table 3. *Hardware Used for Stereotactic Conformation Beam Radiotherapy*

Linac	—Mevatron 77, Siemens, Erlangen, Germany —15 MV X-ray beam used for irradiation
Hardware	—MR-computer: DEC-Micro VAX III —PET-computer: VAX 11/750 DEC —central computer: VAX 3600 —workstation: VAX 3600 —evaluation unit: 8 cpu-multiprocessor system, —Texas Instruments, TMS 320 —host computer: DEC-Micro VAX III —network: DEC-NET
Imaging	—MR Magnetom 63 SP, Siemens, Erlangen, Germany —PET PC-2048-7WB, Scanditronix, Uppsala, Sweden —CT Somatom DRH, Siemens, Erlangen, Germany

Virtual treatment planning: The 3D treatment planning software VOXELPLAN-Heidelberg has been developed at the DKFZ. Determination of the target volume and the organs at risk is assisted by special graphic software tools described in detail elsewhere [7]. An image correlation software package adds the MR and PET information to the conventional CT data on the base of the stereotactic landmarks after correction of geometrical distortions [31]. The geometrical field parameters (isocenter, field size, field form, gantry angle, patient couch rotational angle) can be adjusted while watching the sequences in real-time "beam's eye view"-presentation [9].

Dose calculation: A fast voxel-based real three-dimensional dose calculation algorithm is used based on 3D ray tracing for primary components and 2D convolution for scattering dose. Coplanar and non-coplanar treatment techniques as well as irregular fields can be calculated [10, 11, 34].

Presentation and evaluation of dose distribution: The spatial image information can be displayed in multiplanar reconstructed sections with isodose overlays or as shaded surface images of target volumes, organs at risk and isodoses (3D display) [3, 6]. Quantitative evaluation of 3D dose distribution can be done by dose-volume-histograms and statistical parameter presentation [5, 24].

Transfer of the precalculated isocenter to the patient takes place with the help of a special positioning device mounted onto the wooden base frame and firmly related to the stereotactic co-ordinate system. It has three

Table 2. *Tübingen Arcs*

n	Table	Gantry start	Gantry stop
1	270°	235°	345°
2	300°	235°	345
3	330°	235°	345
4	0°	235°	345
5	0°	15°	125°
6	30°	15°	125°
7	60°	15°	125°

adjustable devices according to the predetermined co-ordinates of the target point [29].

Conformation beam radiotherapy (MLC): Conformation radiotherapy as described by Takahashi [38] means the adaptation of the field to the irregular target volume out of each beam direction. For precision radiotherapy of the head and neck region 3 different-mult-leaf-collimators have been designed in Heidelberg [33]. In daily routine a manual multi-leaf-collimator is used for irradiation with stationary beams or for moving beam treatments with invariable irregular shaped fields [9, 18].

Quality assurance: The immobilization and repositioning accuracy of the head mask has been measured at the DKFZ with an optical sensor system using photogrammetry. This method has been described in detail [27, 33]. Evaluation of the device accuracy includes the determination of the immobilization error and the repositioning error.

3. Patients

3.1. Stereotactic Convergent Beam Radiosurgery

In the first 2 years after clinical use of the SRS 200 system in Tübingen 36 patients with 39 lesions (19 metastases, 11 AVMs, 9 acoustic neurinomas) were treated, 14 male and 12 female with ages ranging from 18 to 79 years (mean age 48, 7 years). This work deals only with the patients with acoustic neurinoma. Until today the follow-up times were 1 to 24 months, with a mean follow-up time of 12, 3 months. Dosage was given according to ICRU to the reference point (mostly corresponding to the isocenter) with the target volume comprising 90% isodose. The first 5 patients with acoustic neurinoma (19–30 mm size) were irradiated with target volume enclosing 16–18 Gy, the maximum dose being 18–23 Gy. In the subsequent treatments the target volume dose was reduced to 12 Gy because of side-effects.

3.2. Stereotactic Conformation Beam Radiotherapy

Gademann *et al.* in 1993 reported the experience of the Heidelberg group with now up to 195 patients and a median follow-up time of 22 months. Details are described in [18]. They describe 3 main types of indications: high-precision radiotherapy (meningioma, low grade glioma, neurinoma, chordoma); boost irradiation to decrease the dose to organs at risk or to achieve an efficient tumour dose; pre-irradiated recurrences.

The group with acoustic neurinoma, which is referred to in this paper, consisted of 12 patients. The follow-up time was 10–40 months (median 28 months), the mean dose administered to the target was 64 Gy in conventional fractions.

III. Results

1. Stereotactic Convergent Beam Radiosurgery

1.1 Dose Distribution

With almost spherical target volumes a very steep dose gradient could be obtained by the 7 standard arcs because of the irradiation of a large spherical sector of the head. The dose gradient of the target volume comprising 90% isodose to 50% isodose was 4 mm to max. 6 mm, almost independent of the collimator. Adaptation of the dose distribution to irregular shaped target volumes was achieved by a combination of several isocenters, individual irradiation arcs and weighting, however, with the drawback of considerable inhomogeneity (Fig. 2, see p. 48) the inhomogeneity over the target volume area was 10–13% for spherical target volumes, 10–25% for oval target volumes, but 25–60% for irregularly shaped target volumes with more than one isocenter.

1.2. Quality Assurance

The best results were obtained in the accuracy of the target point transfer to the stereotaxy unit of the LINAC and the accuracy of the isocenter during moving-field therapy at different gantry and table movements. Measurements during the total quality assurance programme after installation as well as the control measurements with all 39 treatments and different systems resulted in a mechanical isocenter accuracy of 0.3 mm + / − 0.2 mm.

1.3. Time Consumption

The total time needed for fixation, imaging, data handling, hardware application, quality assurance programme and treatment was almost constant for each patient. However, the time needed for treatment planning was very variable and took up to 6 or more hours according to the complexity of the target volume (Table 4).

Table 4. *Time Consumption*

Steps	Convergent radiosurgery	Conformation radiotherapy
Fixation	1/2 hour	1/2 hour
Stereo CT	1 hour	1/2 hour
Stereo MR	—	1 hour
Stereo Angio	1 hour	—
Data handling	1/2 hour	1 hour
Planning	2–4 hours	1/2–3 hours
Application	1/2 hour	1/4 hour
Quality assurance	1 hour	—
Treatment	1/2 hour	1/4 hour per fraction (30)
Mean total time	10 hours	13 hours

1.4. Acoustic Neurinoma

After convergent beam irradiation no further tumour growth was seen in the 9 patients with acoustic neurinoma. Imaging revealed a reduced uptake of contrast medium, particularly in the center. In 4 of 5 patients, who had been irradiated with target volume enclosing 16–18 Gy, side-effects occured. Three patients developed temporary trigeminal paresthesiae 4–9 months after treatment, 1 of them combined with facial paresthesia. This patient showed also a moderate hearing deterioration 8 months after radiosurgery and MR imaging revealed an area of small perifocal oedema. Another patient developed temporary and asymptomatic oedema. Because of those occurrences and the experiences of other groups [Noren, personal communication] the target volume enclosing

dose was reduced to 12 Gy. In the patients, who were treated subsequently with this dose, no side-effects occurred.

2. Stereotactic Conformation Beam Radiotherapy

2.1. Dose Distribution

Using a 3D treatment planning procedure, irregularly shaped fixed fields and non-coplanar irradiation fields, a steep dose gradient at the border of the target volume and almost any adaptation of the dose distribution to irregularly shaped target volumes could be achieved (Fig. 3). Thus, the protection of the surrounding healthy tissue is possible. Only the dose ranges of 10–30% and 30–50% were burdening more of the healthy volume as compared to the convergent beam radiosurgery because of the fixed field irradiation technique.

2.2 Quality Assurance

Results of quality assurance of conformation beam radiotherapy showed that the transfer of the calculated dose to the target point is better than 1 mm [32]. The measured standard deviations of the immobilization accuracy with the DKFZ mask were 0.9 mm anteroposteriorly, 0.7 mm laterally and 1.4 mm inferorsuperiorly. With good patient co-operation an overall immobilization accuracy in the range of $+/-0.2$ mm was achieved [27, 33].

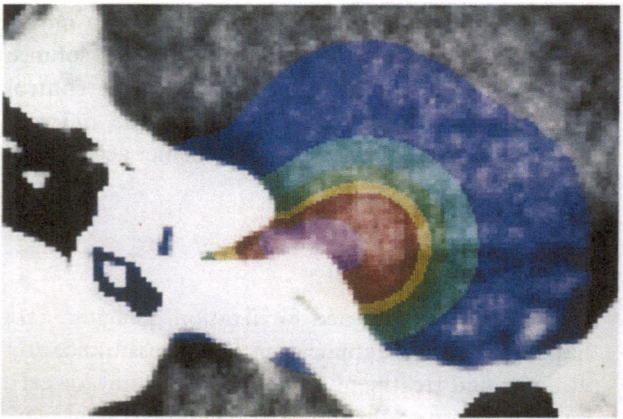

Fig. 2. Dose distribution for Stereotactic Convergent Beam Radiosurgery: acoustic neurinoma with an intrameatal component (mauve 100%–116%, red 90%–100%, yellow 70%–90%, green 50%–70%, light blue 30%–50%, dark blue 10%–30%)

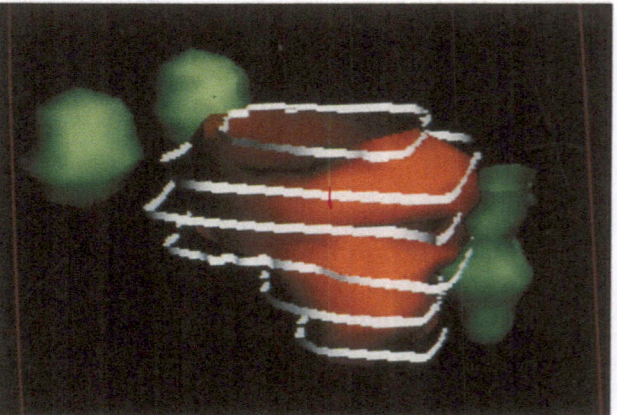

Fig. 3. Dose distribution for Stereotactic Conformation Beam Radiotherapy: three-dimensional shaded surface display of the target volume (red), the 80% isodose (white ribbons) and the organs at risk (eyes and brain stem, green)

2.3. Time Consumption

In the beginning, the new techniques required a total time of up to 10 hours [4]. Increasing experience and optimization of all steps due to new MR imaging sequences, faster hardware and new graphic software tools allowed the reduction of time to 4–5 hours [18] (Table 4).

2.4. Acoustic Neurinoma

Gademann *et al.* report about 12 patients treated by the Heidelberg conformation technique [18]. The follow-up time was a median 28 months, the mean total dose 64 Gy in conventional fractions. Beginning from 3 months after treatment a loss of central uptake of contrast medium was observed in all cases. There were no signs of tumour progression in any patient. Partial response expressing smaller tumour volume in imaging follow-up was seen in 2 patients. In 7 patients no change in tumour size occurred. No side effects such as oedema, facial and trigeminal paresthesiae or hearing deterioration are reported [18].

IV. Discussion

Both stereotactic LINAC based irradiation techniques described in this paper are used in daily clinical routine. Despite many similarities in principles there are great differences in the methods. The Tübingen radiosurgery system is characterized by an isocentric sub-system with a circular secondary collimator. Because of the fixation by screws drilled into the skull this means single dose application, whereas the Heidelberg conformation raditherapy is a combination of conventional fractionated radiotherapy and stereotactic techniques including a mask technique. Radiosurgery achieves a good adaptation of dose distribution to spherical or oval target volumes and a steep dose gradient. However, with the Heidelberg System, using a multi-leaf-collimator for static irradiation techniques, homogeneity and adaptation of the dose distribution to irregularly shaped target volumes by sparing the organs at risk in the immediate vicinity is much better than with radiosurgery, but larger areas of healthy tissue might be subjected to a relatively high dose. By contrast, better results in quality assurance are achieved with the Tübingen convergent beam technique (0.3 mm +/−0.2 mm) as compared to the

Heidelberg conformation beam radiotherapy (< 1 mm). However, there is a limitation by the resolution of the applied imaging techniques.

The price for the high mechanical accuracy of stereotactic single dose application with the Tübingen system is the extended time for the precise adjustment and quality assurance of each patient. However, the Heidelberg system, which is easier to handle, requires a comparable time for the total treatment.

The correct way of treating acoustic neurinomas is still a matter of debate. Problems are arising from the relationship of effect and side-effects. In ou patient population we saw with radiosurgery the same changes in CT/MR follow-up as Gademann *et al.* [18] in their patients treated with fractionated radiotherapy. However, 3 of our first 5 patients developed temporary trigeminal paresthesia, one of them an additional facial paresthesia combined with moderate hearing deterior- ation and a small area of perifocal oedema. Another patient showed asymptomatic oedema. Flickinger 1990 also reported about 85 patients, 28.6% of them developing trigeminal and 30.4% facial neuropathias after radiosurgery [16], whereas Leksell in 1987 described only 15% of 115 patients with temporary facial weakness [23]. However, with fractionated conformation radiotherapy Gademann *et al.* observed no side-effects in their patient population. Future studies will show, whether this method can achieve the same therapeutic effects as radiosurgery (ca. 50% decreased neurinoma, ca. 40% arrested, ca. 10% continued growth [23, 28]) but with less side-effects.

Resulting from these differences in method there are different indication spectra. Radiosurgery is indicated when highest accuracy is clinically required as in the application of a high single dose for AVM [22, 35] or in solitary brain metastasis [13]. Conformation radiotherapy is indicated when from the radiobiological point of view a fractionated irradiation is more effective and mechanically a slightly worse transfer can be accepted (low grade gliomas, meningiomas and others [18]).

Single high dose application does not take advantage of the repair mechanisms in the healthy tissue in contrast to fractionated radiotherapy, thus resulting in a small therapeutic window of radiosurgery.

Further studies will have to determine, which method will bring about the best results of treatment for special indications.

References

1. Bamberg M (1987) Nervensystem. In: Scherer E (ed) Strahlentherapie – Radiologische Onkologie. Springer, Berlin Heidelberg New York Tokyo pp 964–1079
2. Barcia-Salario JL, Hernandez G, Broseta J, Gonzales-Darder J, Ciudad J (1982) Radiosurgical treatment of carotid-cavernous fistula. Appl Neurophysiol 45: 520–522
3. Bauer-Kirpes B, Schlegel W, Boesecke R, Lorenz WJ (1987) Display of organs and isodoses as shaded 3D objects for 3D therapy planning. Int J Radiation Oncol Biol Phys 13: 135–140
4. Becker G, Gademann G, Schlegel W, Lohrum R, Boesecke R, Lorenz WJ (1990) Medical aspects of 3D treatment planning of brain tumours with VOXEL_PLAN Heidelberg. In: Hukku S *et al* (eds) The use of computers in radiotherapy. Proceedings of the Xth International Conference on the use of Computers in Radiation Therapy, Lucknow, pp 147–151
5. Becker G, Lohrum R, Hensley F, Schlegel W, Lyman JT, Weischedel U, Lorenz WJ (1992) Retrospective analysis of complication probabilities induced by radiation treatment of the esophagus. In: Breit (ed) Advanced radiation therapy. Tumour response monitoring and treatment planning. Springer, Berlin Heidelberg New York Tokyo pp 433–440
6. Becker G, Lohrum, R, Werner T, Bürkelbach J, Nemeth G, Boesecke R, Schlegel W, Lorenz WJ (1989) Presentation and evaluation of 3D dose distribution in radiotherapy planning. In: Lemke HU *et al* (eds) Computer assisted radiology. Springer, Berlin Heidelberg New York Tokyo pp 254–261
7. Becker G, Pross J, Bendl R, Mayer G, Lohrum R, Schlegel W (1992) Application of Computer Graphics in 3D Radiotherapy Treatment Planning. In: Breit (ed) Advanced radiation therapy. Tumor response monitoring and treatment planning, pp 561–566
8. Betti OO, Derechinsky V (1983) Irradiation stéréotaxique multifasceaux. Neurochirurgie 29: 295–298
9. Boesecke R, Becker G, Alandt K, Pastyr O, Doll J, Schlegel W, Lorenz WJ (1991) Modification of a three-dimensional treatment planning system for the use of multi-leaf-collimators in conformation radiotherapy. Radiother Oncol 21: 261–268
10. Boesecke R, Doll J, Bauer B, Schlegel W, Pastyr O, Lorenz WJ (1988) Treatment planning for conformation therapy using a multi-leaf-collimator. Strahlentherapie Onkologie 164: 151–154
11. Bortfeld T, Boesecke R, Schlegel W, Bohrung J (1990) 3-D dose calculation using 2-D convolutions and ray tracing methods. In: Hukku S, Iyer PS (eds) The use of computers in radiation therapy. Proceedings of the Xth ICCR, Lucknow, India, Alpana Arts, pp 238–241
12. Colombo F, Benedetti A, Pozza F, Avanzo RC, Marchetti C, Chierego G, Zanardo A (1985) External stereotactic irradiation by linear accelerator. Neurosurgery 16: 154–159
13. Engenhart R, Kimmig B, Höver KH, Wowra B, Romahn J, Lorenz WJ, van Kaick G, Wannenmacher M (1993) Long-term follow-up for brain metastases treated by percutaneous stereotactic single high-dose irradiation. Cancer 71: 1353–1361
14. Engenhart R, Kimmig B, Wowra B, Sturm V, van Kaick G, Wannenmacher M (1989) Stereotaktische Einzeitbestrahlung cerebraler Angiome. Radiologe 29: 219–223
15. Fabrikant JJ, Levy RP, Frankel KA (1989) Stereotactic helium-ion radiosurgery for the treatment of intracranial arteriovenous malformations. In: Heikkingen E *et al* (eds) Proceedings of the International Workshop on Proton and Narrow Photon Beam Therapy, University of Oulu Press, Oulu, pp 33–37
16. Flickinger JC, Lunsford D, Coffey RJ, Linskey ME, Bissonette DJ, Maitz AH, Kondziolka D (1990) Radiosurgery of acoustic neurinomas. Cancer 67: 345–353
17. Friedman WA, Bova FJ (1989) The University of Florida radiosurgery system. Surg Neurol 32: 334–342
18. Gademann G, Schlegel W, Debus J, Schad L, Bortfeld T, Höver KH, Lorenz WJ, Wannenmacher M (1993) Fractionated stereotactically guided radiotherapy of head and neck tumours: a report on clinical use of a new system in 195 cases. Radiother Oncol 29: 205–213
19. Hartmann G, Kimmig B, Treuer H, Bauer B, Lorenz WJ (1987) Treatment planning for convergent beam irradiations in the nasopharynx region. In: Bruinvis *et al* (eds) The use of computers in radiation therapy, I.A.D. Elsevier, North-Holland, pp 349–352
20. Hartmann GH, Schlegel W, Sturm V, Kober B, Pastyr O, Lorenz WJ (1985) Cerebral radiation surgery using moving beam irradiation at a linear accelerator facility. Int J Radiat Oncol Biol Phys 11: 1185–1192
21. Johnson RJ (1975) Radiotherapy of cerebral angiomas with a note on some problems in diagnosis. In: Pia HW *et al* (eds) Cerebral angiomas: advances in diagnosis and therapy. Springer, Berlin Heidelberg New York pp 256–259
22. Kjellberg RN (1986) Stereotactic Bragg peak proton beam radiosurgery for cerebral arteriovenous malformations. Ann Clin Res 18 [Suppl 47]: 17–19
23. Leksell D (1987) Stereotactic radiosurgery. Present status and future trends. Neurol Res 9: 60–68
24. Lohrum R, Becker G, Boesecke R, Werner T, Schlegel W, Lorenz WJ (1992) A medical workstation for the evaluation of alternative 3D radiotherapy treatment plans. Comput Med Imaging Graph 16: 301–309
25. Lutz W, Winston KR, Maleki N (1988) A system for stereotactic radiosurgery with a linear accelerator. Int J Radiation Oncol Biol Phys 14: 373–381
26. Makoski HB, Zeilstra DJ, Nocken U (1988) Arteriovenöse Malformation des Hirnschädels Strahlentherapeutische Aspekte. In: Bamberg M, Sack H (eds) Therapie primärer Hirntumoren. Zuekschwerdt, München, pp 245–249
27. Menke M, Hirschfeld F, Mack T, Pastyr O, Sturm V, Schlegel W (1995) Photogrammetric accuracy measurements of head holder systems used for fractionated radiotherapy. Int J Radiation Oncol Biol Phys, in press
28. Noren G, Arndt J, Hindmarsh T, Hirsch A (1988) Stereotactic radiosurgical treatment of acoustic neurinomas. In: Lunsford LD (ed) Modern stereotactic neurosurgery. Martinus Nijhoff, Boston, pp 481–489
29. Pastyr O, Hartmann GH, Schlegel W, Schabbert S, Treuer H, Lorenz WJ, Sturm V (1989) Stereotactically guided Convergent Beam irradiation with a linear accelerator: localization-technique. Acta Neurochir (Wien) 99: 61–64
30. Podgorsak EB, Olivier A, Pla M, Levebvre P-Y, Hazel P (1988) Dynamic stereotactic radiosurgery. Int J Radiation Oncol Biol Phys 14: 115–126
31. Schad L, Boesecke R, Schlegel W, Hartmann G, Sturm V, Strauss L, Lorenz WJ (1987) Three dimensional image correlation of CT, MR and PET studies in radiotherapy treatment planning of brain tumours. J Comp Ass Tomogr 11: 948–954
32. Schlegel W, Pastyr O, Bortfeld T, Becker G, Schad L, Gademann G, Lorenz WJ (1992) Computer systems and mechanical tools for stereotactically guided conformation therapy with linear accelerators. Int J Radiation Oncol Biol Phys 24: 781–787
33. Schlegel W, Pastyr O, Bortfeld T, Gademann G, Menke M, Maier-Borst W (1993) Stereotactically guided fraction-

ated radiotherapy: technical aspects. Radiother Oncol 29: 197–204

34. Schlegel W, Scharfenberg H, Doll J, Hartmann G, Sturm V, Lorenz WJ (1984) Three dimensional dose planning using tomographic data. In: Cunningham JR (ed) Proceedings of the Eighth International Conference on the Use of Computers in Radiation Therapy, IEEE Computer Society Press, Silver Spring, pp 191–195

35. Steiner L (1988) Stereotactic radiosurgery with the cobalt 60 gamma unit in the surgical treatment of intracranial tumors and arteriovenous malformations. In: Schmidek HH, Sweet WH (eds) Operative neurosurgical techniques, Vol I. Saunders, Philadelphia, pp 515–529

36. Steiner L, Leksell L, Greitz T, Foster DMC, Backlund EO (1972) Stereotaxic radiosurgery for cerebral arteriovenous malformations. Report of a case. Acta Chir Scand 138: 459–464

37. Sturm V, Pastyr O, Schlegel W, Scharfenberg H, Zabel HJ, Netzeband G, Schabbert S, Berberich W (1983) Stereotactic computer tomography with a modified Riechert-Mundinger device as the basis for integrated stereotactic neuroradiological investigations. Acta Neurochir (Wien) 68: 11–17

38. Takahashi S (1965) Conformation radiotherapy: rotation techniques as applied to radiography and radiotherapy of cancer. Acta Radiol [Suppl] 242

Correspondence: Gerd Becker, M.D., Radiotherapy Department, University Hospital, Hoppe-Seyler-Str. 3, D-72076 Tübingen, Federal Republic of Germany.

Acta Neurochir (1995) [Suppl] 63: 52–56

Frameless Stereotaxy for Radiosurgical Planning and Follow-up

M. L. Schwartz, R. Ramani, P. F. O'Brien, C. S. Young, P. Davey, and **P. Hudoba**

Sunnybrook Health Sciences Center, Toronto, Ontario, Canada

Summary

In our centre, 111 patients have been treated with linear accelerator stereotactic radiosurgery. Angiographic, CT and MRI images are generated and the target coordinates calculated in 3 dimensions. For CT scanning, cross sections of perpendicular and oblique fiducial markers are seen.

For follow-up CT scans done without the frame, a virtual frame is generated by means of a computer program that places fiducial markers on each CT scan cut, as if the patient had been wearing the OBT frame and the scan produced with the gantry parallel to the base of the frame. The position of the oblique marker may be calculated by knowing the thickness and position of each CT cut. Various natural fiducial markers (bony landmarks) are identified by coordinates in the scan with the patient wearing the real frame and in the scan with the virtual frame applied. A transformation matrix is utilized to establish the equivalence between the original CT scan with the real frame applied and subsequent scans without the real frame but with the virtual frame applied. In effect, the virtual frame is re-applied in exactly the same position as the real frame.

Lesion measurements may then be duplicated and growth or regression accurately established. The uncertainty in this system of re-application resides in possible patient movement, CT scan slice thickness and inter-observer error in the identification of natural fiducial markers.

Keywords: Radiosurgery; frameless stereotaxy.

Introduction

In our centre, 111 patients; 67 arteriovenous malformations, 34 malignant tumors and 10 acoustic schwannomas, have so far been treated with stereotactic radiosurgery by means of a modified linear accelerator. We have implemented and modified the system originally developed at McGill University. The OBT stereotactic head frame [2] and the McGill dynamic rotation method [4] are used. We began with software commercially available from CMI [3], a version of which is also written for the Leksell stereotactic frame, but have made extensive modifications to it.

The software, which runs on a personal computer, permits the integration of various imaging modalities, digital subtraction angiography (DSA) computed tomography (CT scanning), magnetic resonance imaging (MRI) [1,3]. The software has many functions, allowing the operator to determine the coordinates of any point displayed on a television monitor by positioning the cursor over a structure by means of a mouse. Coronal and sagittal reconstructions may be generated and distances may be measured from one point to another. Additional software, obtained through CMI, but at the time, not commercially available, allows real three-dimensional dose planning for radiosurgery. This software has been extensively modified by one of the authors (RR) so that treatment plans incorporating as many as four isocentres may be made.

At present, there are only three radiosurgery units in Canada. As a result, we receive angiograms and CT and MR images of patients from centres across the country for consideration of radiosurgical treatment. If one is dealing with a lesion with a complex shape or is considering radiosurgical treatment of a lesion in proximity to radiosensitive structures, for example, the optic chiasm or the brain stem, it is useful to be able to make a treatment plan in advance so that radiation distributions are known and appropriate treatment decisions can be made before the patient travels to our centre. In most cases, our patients return home to be followed by the physicians who referred them. It is essential for us to have an accurate method for following lesion size or determining the geographic location of radiation effect as determined by bright signal on T2-weighted magnetic resonance images to treated lesions.

To these ends, we have developed a method by which a virtual frame is applied to CT or MR images acquired in our centre or elsewhere without the stereotactic frame in place. Once the virtual frame has been applied, all the functions of the software developed for treatment planning may then be used with the CT or MR images acquired without the patient wearing the frame.

Methods and Materials

The OBT stereotactic frame which is similar to the Leksell stereotactic frame is applied prior to imaging on the day of radiosurgical treatment and is also used to fix the patient's head to the linear accelerator treatment couch so as to position the patient's lesion at the centre of rotation of both the treatment couch and the linear accelerator gantry which rotate in planes perpendicular to each other. For each imaging modality there is a specific set of fiducial marker plates that attach to the frame. Each CT and MRI fiducial marker plate contains three bars in the shape of an N which, when imaged axially, are seen as three collinear points (Fig. 1). Each CT or MR slice contains nine points derived from the three fiducial marker plates. The coordinate corresponding to the third dimension not seen on the individual CT or MRI slices (y) may be calculated by determining the position of the cross-section of the oblique bar of the N. As shown in Fig. 1, when transverse slices are obtained parallel to the base of the stereotactic frame, the x and z coordinates of the cross-sections of the vertical bars of the N have the same x and z coordinates as they appear in successive transverse CT and MR slices and y is a function of x and the distance between image slices.

When CT or MRI images made without the patient wearing the stereotactic frame are received for analysis, they are first scanned in

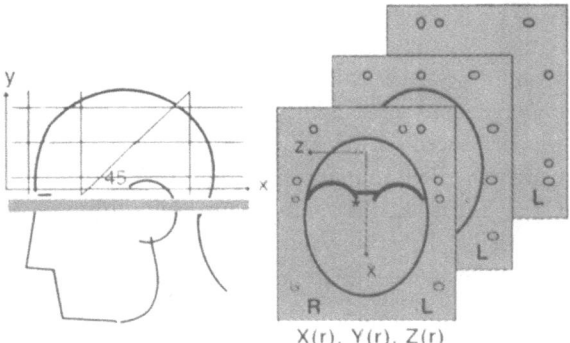

X(r). Y(r). Z(r)

Fig. 1. Frameless stereotaxy: real stereotactic frame (OBT). Each CT and MRI fiducial marker plate contains 3 bars in the shape of an N, which, when imaged axially, are seen as three collinear points. Each CT or MR slice contains 9 points, derived from the three fiducial marker plates. The coordinate corresponding to the third dimension not seen on the individual CT or MRI slices (y) may be calculated by determining the position of the cross-section of the oblique bar on the N. When transverse slices are obtained parallel to the base of the stereotactic frame, the x and z coordinates of the cross-sections of the vertical bars of the N have the same x and z coordinates as they appear in successive transverse CT and MR slices and y is a function of x and the distance between the image slices

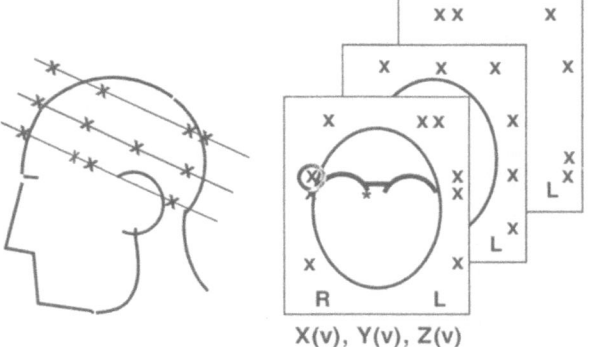

X(v), Y(v), Z(v)

Fig. 2. Frameless stereotaxy: virtual frame. A virtual frame is generated with an arbitrary starting point, the cross-section of a vertical marker, as indicated by the circled X. This marker may be placed anywhere and need not be outside the patient's head. The position of the other vertical markers is automatically determined by choosing the starting point because the cross-sectional appearance of the stereotactic frame is known and the scale of the image has been measured. In effect, the other vertical markers are placed as though the scan had been made with the patient wearing a stereotactic frame with the CT or MR image plane parallel to the base of the frame

an analogue to digital scanner and then converted to the format required by the CMI program by means of software written by one of the authors (RR). These images are transferred to the image directory where they are available to the CMI program so that they then may be viewed on the television monitor. The first transaxial image is then assessed and its magnification determined by measuring the five-centimetre scale provided by the CT or MR scanner. The offset distance of each subsequent CT or MRI slice is acquired. In this way, the distance between each cross-section is known. It is assumed that there is no movement of the patient during the acquisition of image slices so that the offset distances indicated by the scanner truly represent the distance between real anatomical features shown slice by slice.

A virtual frame is then generated with an arbitrary starting point, the cross-section of a vertical marker as indicated in Fig. 2 by the circled x. This marker may be placed anywhere and need not be outside the patient's head. The position of the other vertical markers is automatically determined by choosing the starting point because the cross-sectional appearance of the stereotactic frame is known and the scale of the image has been measured. In effect, the other vertical markers are placed as though the scan had been made with the patient wearing a stereotactic frame with the CT or MR image plane parallel to the base of the frame. The position of the cross-section of the oblique bar of the N may then also be displayed because the offset of each transverse slice is known. Partial correction for patient movement or malregistration of images digitized by the scanner is achieved by manually aligning structures known to have a regular contour as shown in Figs. 3 and 4.

Various natural fiducial markers are then selected. The anterior clinoid process (as indicated in Fig. 5), the apex of the internal auditory canal and the promontory of the inner ear have proved most useful. Since all geometric functions of the CMI software apply, coronal and sagittal reconstructions may be made. The alternate views are helpful to refine the choice of the best locus of the selected natural fiducial marker. Three views of each selected natural fiducial marker are obtained and the best coordinates of the selected point determined using the software and the arbitrarily-placed virtual

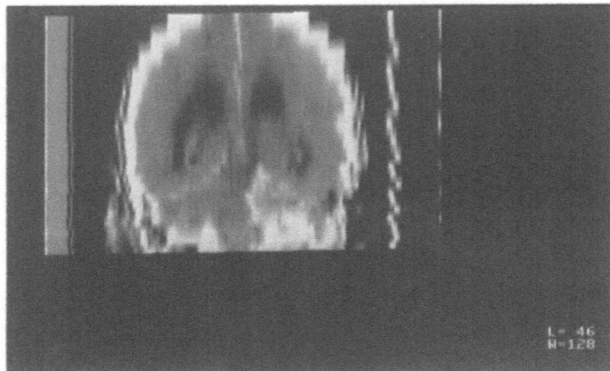

Fig. 3. A coronal reconstruction of the CT scan of a patient with a left recurrent acoustic neuroma is shown. The skull vault has an irregular contour because of patient movement or malregistration of images digitized by the analogue to digital scanner

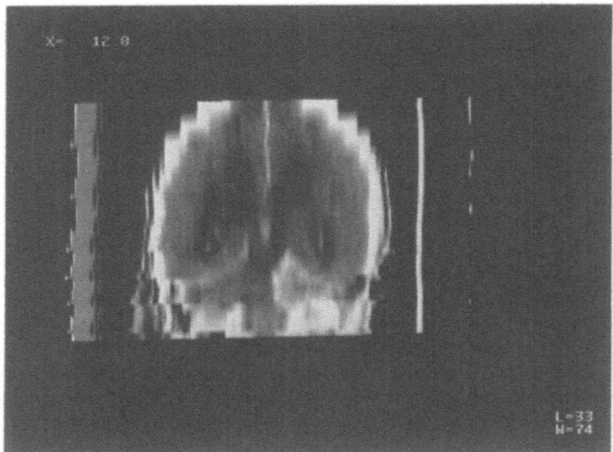

Fig. 4. Manual correction has smoothed the contour of the left parietal bone which is known to be smooth

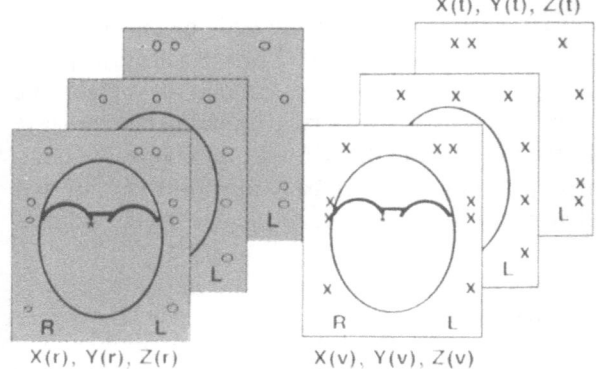

Fig. 5. Frameless stereotaxy: transformed coordinates. The anterior clinoid process, as indicated by the asterisk may be chosen as a natural fiducial marker. Three views of each selected natural fiducial marker are obtained. The coordinates of equivalent points identified in the real and virtual frames are designated (r) and (v) respectively. Transformed coordinates (t) may be compared with x(r), y(r), z(r)

with respect to the patient's head. The error in this system of transformation resides in CT or MRI scan slice thickness, interobserver error in the identification of natural and frame fiducial markers and movement of the patient in the CT or MRI scanner at the time of the study done without the real stereotactic frame. This error has been measured.

Results

The effect of slice thickness on the accuracy of the identification of bony landmarks as natural fiducial markers is significant. The first study was done with the patient wearing the stereotactic frame to evacuate a tumor cyst. A second study, done for further patient management without the stereotactic frame in place was produced with 5 millimetre-thick CT scan slices. Care was taken to immobilize the patient's head in the CT scanner so that movement between slices was impossible. Four bony anatomical points easily seen in the studies done with and without the real stereotactic frame were selected and the transformation method applied. No coronal or sagittal reconstructions were used. The measurement errors were determined and the contributions of the x, y and z error vectors to the total error were determined. The standard deviations were $x = 2.8$ mm, $y = 5.53$ mm and $z = 2.23$ millimetres.

As part of a protocol to measure the change in apparent size of cerebral metastases after a delay following the injection of iodinated contrast material, two separate CT scans utilizing 1 mm slices were made 40 minutes apart with a patient wearing the stereotactic frame. The first study was made with the CT gantry

frame. The coordinates of selected fiducial marker indicated in Fig. 5 are given as x(v), y(v) and z(v).

The same natural fiducial markers are then imaged and their coordinates determined in another CT or MRI scan, done with the patient actually wearing the OBT frame. The coordinates with the patient wearing the real frame are given as x(r), y(r) and z(r) in Fig. 5. Because the position of the real frame with respect to the patient's head is different from that of the virtual frame, the coordinates given by the CMI program for a particular landmark are different from those given for the virtual frame applied to the CT or MRI study.

As the real and virtual frames have the same size and shape, the coordinates for any recognizable landmark in one study are related to those of the equivalent point in the other study, as though translation and rotation of the same frame had occurred between studies. As a result, using a transformation matrix and any three equivalent points, the coordinates for any point on the display of any CT or MRI slice, as given by x(v), y(v) and z(v), may be transformed to x(t), y(t) and z(t). Conceptually, the transformation matrix translates and rotates the virtual frame to the same position as the real frame (image plane) parallel to the base of the OBT frame and the second with the frame deliberately placed at an angle to the CT image plane. The coordinates of the natural fiducial markers (anatomical landmarks) with respect to the stereotactic frame which had not moved relative to the patient's head would be expected to be the same in both studies although the appearance of the CT slices was quite different because of change in the position of the patient's head (and stereotactic frame) with respect to the CT scan image plane. Any difference in coordinates represents the error in identifying the same bony landmark in different CT scans. It was impossible to reliably identify the same point on the promontory of the inner ear in the two studies because of the different CT angle but the centre of the clinoid process and the apex of the internal auditory meatus proved resistant to translation and rotation with respect to the CT image plane. The error attributable to the uncertainty in identifying the anatomical landmarks was (standard deviations) $x = 0.43$ mm, $y = 0.71$ mm and $z = 0.43$ mm. The computation error, that is, the residual error after subtracting the anatomical landmark error was negligible. The pixel size of our display system (software and hardware) is 0.67 millimetres.

Discussion

Figure 6 shows a sagittal reconstruction through the right anterior clinoid process in a patient with an acoustic neuroma. The cursor has been placed at the mid-point of the anterior clinoid process in its vertical dimension. Utilization of the coronal or sagittal reconstructions allows the observer to choose the locus of a bony landmark more reliably than if the reconstructions were not available.

Figure 7 shows a malignant astrocytoma, recurrent after partial surgical resection and conventional fractionated external beam photon irradiation. The patient was referred for consideration of palliative treatment using conformal radiosurgery. As the tumor is close to the optic nerve and as the development of a treatment plan with several isocentres may be complex and time-consuming, the virtual frame was applied to the CT scan done at another hospital and the radiation isodose contours indicated in Fig. 7 was produced. It was elected to treat the patient. The actual treatment plan utilized is indicated in Fig. 8. None of the nine coordinates specifying the three treatment isocentres had to be changed by more than two millimetres in

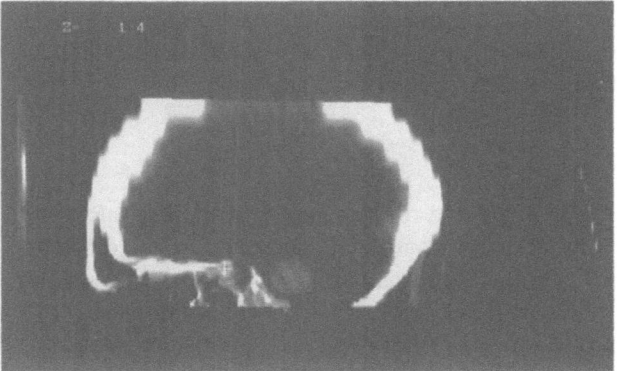

Fig. 6. The cursor has been placed at the midpoint of the anterior clinoid process as seen in the sagittal reconstruction through the right anterior clinoid process in a patient with an acoustic neuroma. Utilization of the coronal or sagittal reconstructions allows the observer to choose the locus of a bony landmark more reliably than if the reconstructions were not available

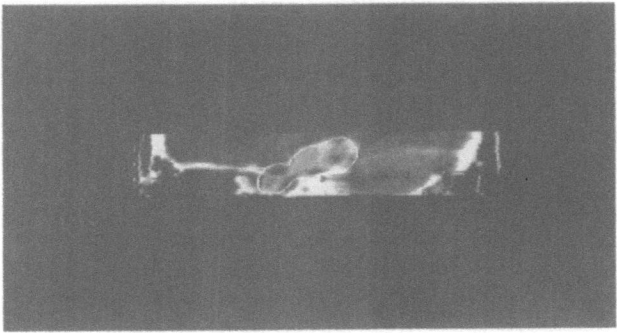

Fig. 7. The sagittal reconstruction of a CT scan done at another hospital without a stereotactic frame in place is illustrated. A treatment plan with 3 isocentres was made by applying the virtual frame to the CT scan and using the radiosurgery planning software

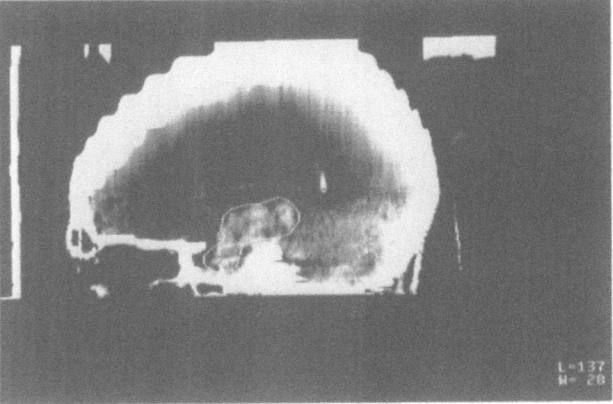

Fig. 8. The actual treatment plan used for this patient produced with him wearing the real stereotactic frame is illustrated. None of the 9 coordinates specifying the 3 treatment isocentres had to be changed by more than 2 millimetres

converting the treatment plan derived from the CT scan done at another hospital without the stereotactic frame to the treatment plan actually used.

Conclusion

The error due to uncertainty in finding the same bony landmarks (natural fiducial markers) in different CT studies depends in part on slice thickness and is as little as 0.43 in 1 mm slices. The computational error is negligible. The potential error caused by patient movement between slices cannot be quantified but may be recognized and partially compensated for. This method of frameless stereotaxy has proved useful in radiosurgical planning and follow-up.

References

1. Henri CJ, Collins DL, Peters TM (1991) Multimodality image integration for stereotactic surgical planning. Med Phys 18(2): 167–177
2. Olivier A, Bertrand G (1982) Stereotaxic device for percutaneous twist-drill insertion of depth electrodes and for brain biopsy. J Neurosurg 56: 307–308
3. Peters TM, Clark JA, Olivier A, Marchand EP, Mawko G, Dieumegarde M, Muresan LV, Eng M, Ethier R (1986) Integrated stereotaxic imaging with CT, MR imaging, and digital subtraction angiography. Radiology 161(3): 821–826
4. Podgorsak EB, Olivier A, Pla M, Lefebvre P, Hazel J (1988) Dynamic stereotactic radiosurgery. Int J Radiat Oncol Biol Phys 14: 115–125

Correspondence: Michael L. Schwartz, M.D., Sunnybrook Health Sci. Center, 2075 Bayview Av., Suite A129, Toronto, Ontario, M4N, 3M5, Canada.

Acta Neurochir (1995) [Suppl] 63: 57–59
© Springer-Verlag 1995

Stereotactic Radiotherapy for AVMs: The University of Toronto Experience

C. S. Young, M. L. Schwartz, P. O'Brien, and **R. Ramaseshan**

Toronto-Sunnybrook Regional Cancer Centre, Sunnybrook Health Sciences Centre, The University of Toronto Brain Vascular Malformation Study Group, Toronto, Ontario, Canada

Summary

Since July 1989, 66 patients have received stereotactic radiosurgery for arteriovenous malformations of the brain. All cases were reviewed by our multidisciplinary group. As result of our treatment algorithms these patients underwent stereotactic radiosurgery, either as the sole therapy or as part of combined modality treatment. Using a 6 MV linear accelerator, we have usually employed doses of either 15 or 20 Gy to the edge of the lesion, ensuring that critical normal structures do not receive a dose in excess of 15 Gy. Of the initial 24 patients followed for a minimum of 2 years, 12 have complete obliteration documented by angiography; 8 have > 90% obliteration (several have deferred further angiographic follow-up which may show progression to complete obliteration); 3 have had the nidus diminish; and one has had no change. Within this cohort, one patient experienced a transient acute effect; one patient has developed a minor late effect; one suffered a fatal hemorrhage despite ongoing response to radiosurgery; one has recently undergone retreatment.

Keywords: Stereotactic radiosurgery; AVM; linac.

Introduction

Since its development over 40 years ago, radiosurgery has been used for a variety of intracranial disorders, including arteriovenous malformations. However, its role in the management of AVMs continues to be better defined as more experience accumulates world-wide.

The University of Toronto Brain Vascular Malformation Study Group is a multi-disciplinary group comprised of one radiation oncologist, two interventional neuroradiologists and three neurosurgeons. With these three disciplines, we are able to offer stereotactic radiosurgery, embolization and surgery for patients with brain AVMs. We receive consultations both locally and from across Canada.

Since July 1989, we have been able to provide stereotactic radiosurgery. We have now treated 66 patients, with 24 eligible (as of August 31, 1993) for a minimum follow-up of 2 years. The results of this initial group of patients is presented.

Patient Selection

Our multi-disciplinary group has developed treatment algorithms which incorporate our opinions regarding hemorrhagic risk plus our desire to involve patients in decision-making. The algorithms are briefly outlined below:

Unless patients are very elderly (when the 4% annual risk of hemorrhage compounded out over the remainder of their expected lifespan is low) or have other more immediate life-threatening diseases, we recommend treatment (if technically feasible and with acceptable morbidity) for all patients.

For those with a recent hemorrhage, we feel the risk of re-hemorrhage is significant enough within the first several years to warrant pursuing a therapy which can confer immediate protection. Thus, patients are considered first for surgery plus or minus embolization. Occasionally, embolization will obliterate the lesion, obviating other therapy. If these modalities are not feasible, or do not result in complete obliteration, or are not acceptable to the patient, then stereotactic radiotherapy (for lesions less than 3.0 cm) is an option.

For those without a recent hemorrhage and no need for immediate obliteration of the AVM (such as a rapidly progressing neurological deficit), then a therapy with a potential latency period of several years is an acceptable option. For patients with lesions less than 3.0 cm, stereotactic radiotherapy (plus or minus embolization) is considered first by our group. However, patients are informed embolization alone can occasionally obliterate the lesion, and surgery may also be technically feasible. The patients then decide, based upon their desire to avoid an invasive surgical procedure versus their acceptance of a delayed obliteration with the attendant risk of a hemorrhage during that latency period. It has been interesting to observe the heterogeneity of responses to these relative risks.

Method

Following the application of an OBT headframe, angiography, CT plus or minus MR imaging are obtained. Using the McGill system, planning ensues with the ability to visualize the isodose distributions on all forms of imaging. With a 6 MV linear accelerator, the radiation is delivered via the McGill system of dynamic rotation. Removing the flattening filter increases the output such that the beam on-time is on the order of five minutes.

Data regarding the dose-response of both AVMs and eloquent normal tissue are not available. To try to elucidate this, we have employed only two minimum target doses (the first few patients were treated to 25 Gy) while adhering to the following:

1. Either 15 or 20 Gy is prescribed as the minimum target dose. (Two of the early patients received 25 Gy as the minimum target dose.)
2. Eloquent normal tissue receives a maximum of 15 Gy.
3. The isodose line encompassing the edge of the target may vary from 50% to 90%, provided above criteria are met. Commonly, the 90% isodose is the minimum target isodose.
4. Multiple isocentres may be used.

Ideally, imaging follow-up consists of annual MR scans, with angiography to confirm any MR evidence of complete obliteration. Given that patients are referred from across our country, the variable access to such imaging coupled with the reluctance of some to undergo repeat angiography results in less than complete information than desired. The criteria employed by our neuroradiologists for complete obliteration are stringent and defined as the absence of both the nidus and any evidence of AV shunting, such as an early draining vein. For those unable to be followed with MR (i.e., due to intracranial clip), angiography beginning at least at two years is requested.

Results of 24 Patients

A. Patient Characteristics

1. Sex	Male	14
	Female	10
2. Age at treatment:	< 20 yrs	1
	20–40 yrs	15
	40–60 yrs	5
	> 60 yrs	3
3. Prior treatment:	none	9
	surg + embo	4
	embo	11
4. Prior hemorrhage:	yes	15
	no	9

B. Treatment

Minimum target dose:	25 Gy	2
	20 Gy	16
	15 Gy	6
Length of follow-up:	2–3 yrs	17
	3–4 yrs	6
	> 4 yrs	1

C. Outcome

1. Angio confirmed oblit	11
Only MRI confirmed oblit	1
Near total oblit	9
Nidus smaller	3
No change	1

2. Minimum target dose	Oblit	Nearly oblit
25 Gy	1	1
20 Gy	7	9
15 Gy	3	
	Smaller	No change
25 Gy	2	1

3. Size	Oblit	Nearly oblit
< 1 cm	2	1
< 2 cm	10	5
< 3 cm		1
> 3 cm		
	Smaller	No change
< 1 cm	1	
< 2 cm	3	1

4. Acute effects	1
Late effects	1
Hemorrhage	1
Death from hemorrhage	1

Discussion

With our treatment algorithms, the number of patients receiving stereotactic radiosurgery is small. Difficulties in obtaining timely follow-up imaging (several with previously documented nearly complete obliteration have delayed their scheduled follow-up angiography) impede a full current assessment of their outcome.

Given these constraints, no definite dose-response or size effect can be demonstrated. The patient without a documented response at 1 year, received a minimum 15 Gy to an AVM replacing the posterior portion of his corpus callosum. Treated with multiple isocentres, it was well tolerated. However, it is not surprising that no early response is seen. Due to an aneurysmal clip, MR imaging is excluded, and the patient has deferred further follow-up until 3 years.

With respect to acute effects, 1 patient experienced transient dysphasia within 8 hours following treatment. Hemorrhage was excluded. Her symptoms resolved within 36 hours, and have never recurred.

Our only patient with a late effect developed a minor difficulty balancing on one leg approximately 18 months post treatment. This has remained stable; the nidus is obliterated; but a small early vein persisted at 2 years, resulting in an observation of near total obliteration. This may well resolve by the third year.

One patient, aged 25, had a 1 cm retrothalamic AVM treated to a minimum target dose of 20 Gy. Although 1 and 2 year MR imaging showed progressive diminution in the size of the nidus, she unfortunately suffered a fatal hemorrhage at 2.5 years post treatment. Interestingly, two patients have resolution of all but a small dural-based component. Given the expertise within our group, these patients will be offered embolization to, hopefully, effect a complete obliteration.

One patient still had evidence of a small, early draining vein (nidus not visualized) at 3 years. Given the response to radiation, but acknowledging that further time was unlikely to result in complete obliteration, she underwent retreatment recently.

Conclusions

1. Assessment is hampered by difficulties in securing timely follow-up imaging. More time is required to determine if our outcome (currently with 12 documented obliterations, plus the 8 near total obliterations) will be similar to that of other series.
2. Similarly, our numbers are too small and our data incomplete to allow any conclusions regarding dose and response. While some may postulate that lower doses will require a longer period for obliteration, three patients treated with a minimum target dose of 15 Gy to lesions from 1.25 to 2.5 cm, attained complete obliteration within 2 years.
3. The doses employed resulted in an acceptable morbidity with acute and late effects developing in only 1/24 respectively.
4. Unfortunately, our experience underscores the need for complete obliteration to protect from recurrent hemorrhage, with one patient suffering a fatal hemorrhage despite ongoing response to radiation.

References

1. Steiner L, Lindquist C, Adler JR, Torner JC, Alves W, Stein M (1992) Clinical outcome of radiosurgery for cerebral arteriovenous malformations. J Neurosurg 77: 1–8.
2. Friedman WA, Bova FJ (1992) Linear accelerator radiosurgery for arteriovenous malformation. J Neurosurg 77: 832–841
3. Colombo F, Benedetti A, Possa F, Marchetti C, Chierego G (1989) Linear accelerator radiosurgery of cerebral arteriovenous malformations. Neurosurgery 24: 833–840
4. Betti OO, Munari C, Rosler R (1989) Stereotactic radiosurgery with the linear accelerator: Treatment of arteriovenous malformations. Neurosurgery 24: 311–321.
5. Lunsford LD, Kondziolka D, Flickinger JC, Bissonette DJ, Jungreis CA, Maitz AH, Horton JA, Coffey RJ (1991) Stereotactic radiosurgery for arteriovenous malformations of the brain. J Neurosurg 75: 512–525.
6. Sutcliffe JC, Forster DMC, Walton L, Dias PS, Kemeny AA (1992) Untoward clinical effects after stereotactic radiosurgery for intracranial arteriovenous malformations. Br J Neurosurg 6: 177–185

Correspondence: Charlene Young, M.D., F.R.C.P.C., Department of Radiation Oncology, Toronto-Sunnybrook Regional Cancer Center, 2075 Bayview Avenue, Toronto, Ontario M4N3M5, Canada.

Acta Neurochir (1995) [Suppl] 63: 60–67

Radiosurgery in the Treatment of Cerebral AVMs

D. I. Levy, K. Kitz, M. Killer, and **B. Richling**

Department of Neurosurgery, University of Vienna Medical School, Wien, Austria

Summary

Radiosurgery of AVM's is gaining in popularity and is advocated by many for the treatment of lesions less than 3 cm in diameter. During a 17 month period 33 patients with cerebral AVM's were treated with radiosurgery. All regions of the brain were represented in the series including brain stem. A mean follow-up of 10.8 months revealed a 6% rebleed rate and a 9% total complication rate. Multimodality therapy including embolization and surgery is recommended for the treatment of AVM's and radiosurgery is seen as an important adjunctive treatment option.

Keywords: Radiosurgery; arteriovenous malformations; gamma knife.

Introduction

The Treatment of intracranial arteriovenous malformations has rapidly developed in the last decade. What was once primarily a surgical therapeutic approach now uses embolization and stereotactic radiosurgery both primarily and in combination. The systems which have been extensively used for radio-surgery include proton radiosurgery [11, 12], multiple cobalt-60 beams (the "gamma knife") [26], linear accelerator-based radiosurgery [2, 3] and helium ion radiosurgery [25].

Laboratory studies have shown that single large doses of radiation to the brain produce localized endothelial proliferation [31]. Thus, the mechanism responsible for the response of AVMs to any of the radiosurgical systems appears to be the induction of localized endothelial cell proliferation, vascular wall thickening, and thrombosis of the malformation [14]. Radiosurgery has been advocated mainly for AVMs less than 3 centimeters in greatest diameter, as the larger lesions have poorer results both for size reduction and radiation damage risk [12, 13, 16]. We have

seen promising results from radiosurgery in our patient population, where gamma knife radiosurgery is used primarily as an adjuvant to embolization and surgery.

Patients and Methods

Between August 1992 and December 1993, 33 patients with cerebral AVMs were treated using a gamma knife (Leksell Inc. Stockholm, Sweden) at the University of Vienna. The group consisted of 18 men and 15 women with an average age of 39.5 years (range 16–79 years). The AVMs were distributed as seen in Table 1, with the greatest frequency in thalamic, fronto-parietal, and brainstem locations. The sizes of the AVMs are recorded in Table 2 with a relatively even distribution of small, medium and large AVMs.

Most of the patients (28 of 33) had endovascular glue embolization prior to gamma knife therapy. The ability to successfully embolize the AVM depends on several factors that are beyond the scope of this paper. In the largest number of cases the AVM could be embolized to an 80–99% reduction in nidus. The percentage reduction of nidus is shown in Table 3.

All patients had application of the Leksell stereotactic frame and underwent their pre-gamma knife treatment under local anaesthesia supplemented by intravenous sedation. The various stereotactic studies used for lacalization included cerebral angiography, stereotactic MRI and in 40% of patients, CT angiography. Biplane stereotactic angiograms were obtained to define the AVM nidus and determine the target co-ordinates. In all cases angiographic co-ordinates and selected isodose lines were superimposed on stereotactic MRI images to detect critical areas. In 40% of patients a stereotactic CT angiography was performed and compared with data of angiography and MRI.

The mean dose delivered to the AVM margin was 17.3 Gy (range 12 to 24 Gy), and that delivered to the center of the AVM was 35.5 Gy (range 28 to 50 Gy). A peripheral dose line of 50% or greater was utilized in 77.9% of patients.

The average clinical follow-up was 10.8 months which unfortunately includes angiographic follow-up on very few patients. We have included permanent (> 6 weeks) complications following both embolization and gamma knife therapy. Symptoms of drowsiness, vomiting and sensory disturbances of short duration were expected and not reported as complications of therapy.

Three patients also underwent surgery after embolization and before gamma knife therapy. These three patients were the only ones

Table 1

Location of AVMs ($n = 33$)	
Thalamic	7
Frontoparietal	6
Brainstem	5
Corpus callosum	3
Parietal	3
Frontal	2
Occipital	2
Temporal	2
Cerebellar	2
Basal ganglia	1

Table 2. *Size of AVM in Greatest Diameter*

Size of AVM	
< 2 cm	13 (40%)
2–4 cm	11 (33%)
> 4 cm	9 (27%)

Table 3. *Percentage of AVM Embolized with Glue Prior to Radiosurgery*

% Embolization	
< 50%	7
50–79%	9
80–99%	10
100%	2

in our study to receive all three modalities currently accepted for AVM treatment.

Results

The follow-up after gamma knife therapy is too short to make conclusive statements about efficacy in the treatment of cerebral AVMs. However we can report on short term rebleedings and complications (Table 4). The only complication of embolization seen in this group was a left hemiparesis from glue embolization of a large right precentral AVM.

Complications after gamma knife surgery thus far includes three patients (9%). There were 2 rebleedings, one 6 months after gamma knife radiation following embolization of a medium sized (2–4 cm) thalamic AVM. The second occurred 1 year after embolization and gamma knife radiation to a large (> 4 cm) corpus

Table 4. *Complications After Gamma Knife Therapy*

Rebleed	2 (6%)
Hemisensory disturbance	1 (3%)
Total	3 (9%)

callosum AVM. Neither of the bleeds were associated with neurological deficit.

Discussion

The principle objective in treating an AVM is angiographic obliteration with minimal patient risk. Surgical excision gives immediate protection but in some cases, the size or location of the AVM precludes surgery [7]. In radiosurgery the therepeautically effective radiation dose is delivered in a single session whereas in radiotherapy the radiation is given in fractions. The advantages of radiosurgery as well as its disadvantages are becoming well established [6]. The results of cerebral AVM treatments have been particularly rewarding and the adverse clinical effects are improving as more experience accumulates. In gamma knife surgery of cerebral AVMs an 80–87% obliteration rate is claimed in the best series [13, 26] with permanent adverse clinical effects between 3 and 9%.

All radiosurgical methods used depend on thrombosing an AVM primarily as a function of size, geometry, and radiation dose. The incidence of obliteration increases with an increase in minimum AVM margin radiation dose. The risk of deficit also rises as the margin dose is increased.

Adverse effects of radiation have been seen on CT and now more commonly on MRI. Although MRI is more sensitive than CT for detecting pathologic changes in the central nervous system, it can still not differentiate between radiation injury, postoperative change, post-haemorrhagic change and gliotic brain tissue. Histologically, an AVM is a cluster of pathological vessels and intervening non-viable brain tissue [20]. The increased signal seen on MRI post gamma knife is most probably due to damage of the pathologic vessels with blood brain barrier breakdown. It could also be radiation injury to the intervening non-viable brain tissue or a combination of both mechanisms [14].

Due to the delayed action of radiosurgery, the patient is at risk for bleeding until the AVM is completely thrombosed, which will not occur in 13–24% of cases in the best series [3, 12, 15, 25]. Haemorrhage has not been observed in any patient once angiography has confirmed complete obliteration; however, haemorrhage has been reported even after a 95% reduction in size following radiosurgery [25]. The risk of incomplete obliteration and delayed radiation induced neuronal damage is greatest for AVMs, larger than 3 cm in diameter [3, 12, 15]. Larger AVMs can be treated, but for comparable obliteration rates, radiosurgery involves a higher brain injury risk [30].

The gamma knife series by Steiner *et al.* includes 326 AVM patients [29]. Following radiation, the risk of rebleeding was 2% per year, neurological deficits occurred in 3% and residual AVMs, were seen in between 16% and 21% of patients followed for 2 years or more. In Lundsford's series of 227 AVM patients, neurological deficits were seen in 6.7%, rebleeding was seen in 4%, and 24% of patients had residual AVMs at 2 year follow-up [15].

The latency period for radiosurgical treatment effecting obliteration of an AVM is estimated to be 1 to 2 years or more [28]. With the introduction of MRI follow-up, abscence of flow voids have prompted some to angiogram earlier demonstrating some AVMs obliterated before 1 year [29].

Adverse Effects of Radiosurgery

After gamma knife therapy, neurological deficits are not uncommon. Steiner *et al.* report neurological outcomes in 228 patients with a mean follow-up of 7 years [27] After radiosurgery, chronic headache occurred in 43% of patients of which 34% of these persisted. Motor deficit occurred in 33% with 45% of these persisting. Seizures occurred in 26% of cases with 59% persisting. Memory problems were reported by 19% of patients and language disturbance was described in 15% of cases.

There continues to be speculation that radiosurgery is overused in regard to the primary treatment of what are considered surgical AVMs [24, 30]. This occurs with many new methods where expensive equipment and a potential for a better, safer procedure exists. There are currently at least 12 gamma knife centers and more than 100 linear accelerator centers in the United States. Enthusiasm and inexperience may unduly expand indications as the field rapidly grows and more data are gathered [30].

There is no doubt that superficial AVMs, even in eloquent areas can be surgically extirpated with low risk [24]. However, there are patients and even neurosurgeons who will not agree to open surgery in even low risk cases. Therefore radiosurgery has been used and will continue to be used on patients that would achieve with lower risk a certain post-operative cure with open surgery.

Tumour Induction Following Radiosurgery

Tumours have been induced by radiotherapy in both low and high doses. Radiosurgery on the other hand, has induced no reported tumours in the 25 years since its introduction. It has been speculated that ionizing beams delivered over a long period are more prone to induce tumour development than a single high dose given over a short period [30]. This observation however, does not exclude the possibility of future tumour cases linked to radiosurgery.

Radiosurgery and Growth Hormone Deficit

Following fractionated radiation therapy growth hormone deficit is observed in 30% of children. In Steiner *et al.* series of 126 children between 3 and 2 years of age treated with gamma knife radiosurgery, no growth hormone deficit was observed. This result is hypothesized to be due to the relatively small tissue volumes targeted, sparing the hypothalamus [30].

Further Therapy After Unsuccessful Radiosurgery

Obliteration rate is dependent on initial AVM size, with smaller AVMs showing a better rate of reduction [12]. The 24 and 36 month follow-up usually shows progression of the process. However, significant thrombosis has not been observed past the 36 month angiogram, and thrombosis has not been observed to begin after 24 months [25]. Therefore, if there has been no change in AVM architecture at 24 months, or if obliteration has not been observed at 36 months, alternative treatment is recommended [19]. Surgical treatment, further embolization or further radiosurgery are all possibilities. It has been suggested that prior radiosurgery did not present problems for further endovascular treatment and appeared to make surgery easier. Three AVMs were surgically resected after unsuccessful radiosurgery and the vessels were observed by the operating surgeon to be easier to manipulate and cauterize than unradiated AVMs [19]. In patients who are referred following prior unsuccessful radiosurgery, there is benefit to further reducing the nidus prior to repeat treatment. The delayed adverse reactions of focused radiation are thought to be dose-volume related and thus embolization may be helpful in further reducing the target volume, minimizing the cumulative radiation dose to adjacent normal tissue. There appears to be no increased risk of subsequent embolization and endovascular procedures in a small series of 6 radiosurgically treated AVMs. However, due to the known histological changes of radiosurgery including stenosis and occlusion of feeding vessels, a damaged intima, frayed elastic membrane and medial muscle necrosis, caution is recommended as such vessels would be prone to dissection [19].

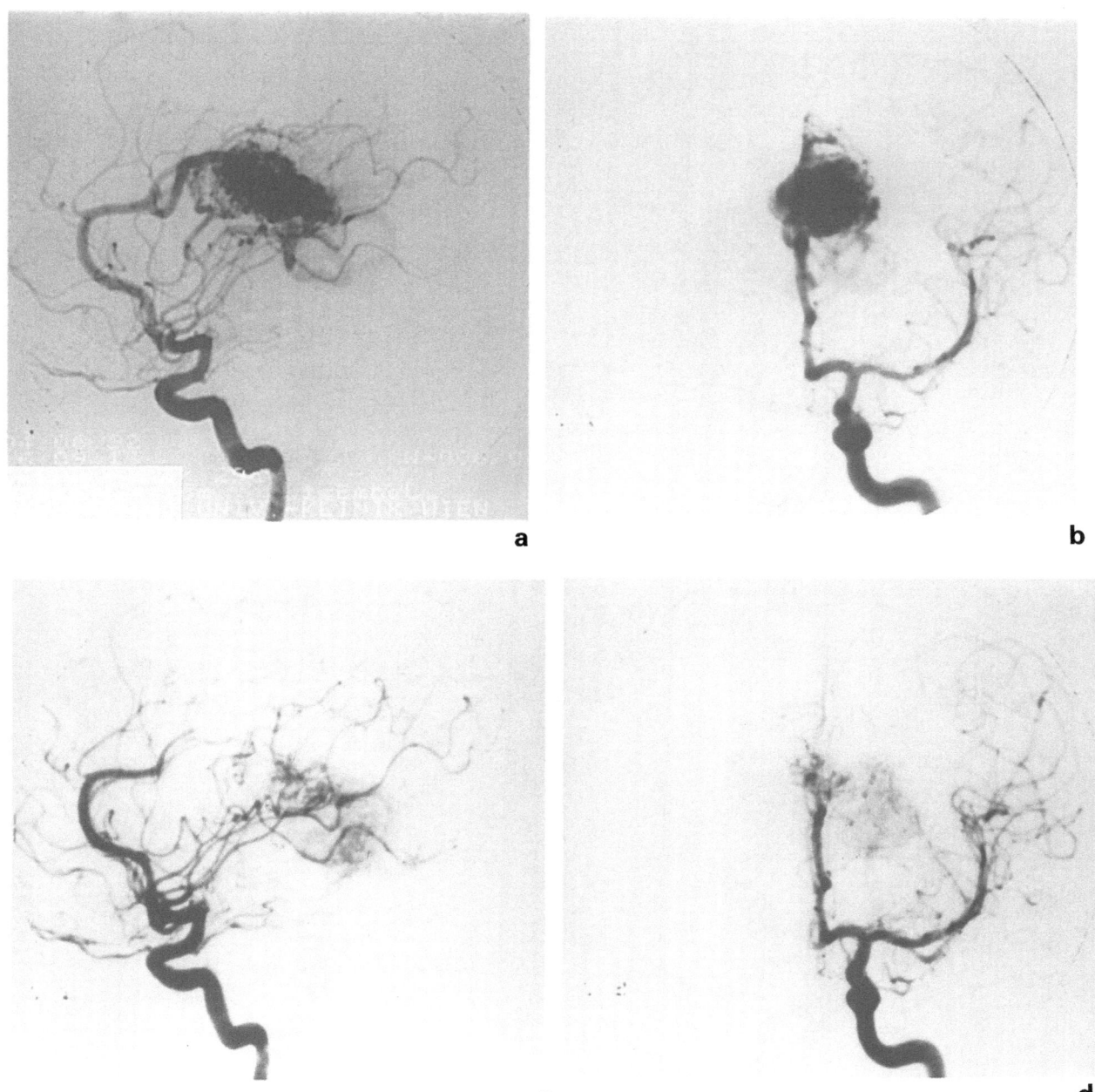

Fig. 1. 29 year old patient with corpus callosum AVM. (a, b) Left ICA pre-embolization AP + lateral projections. (c, d) Left ICA post-embolization AP + lateral

Associated Aneurysms

Both radiosurgery [30] and embolization of AVMs [18, 19] claim to be effective methods of thrombosing intranidal and flow related aneurysms, thus reducing the risk of subsequent haemorrhage. However, because of the increased risk of haemorrhage with associated aneurysms in an AVM patient, we recommend surgical or endovascular treatment to immediately eliminate the risk of aneursymal bleeding.

The Role of MRI in Radiosurgery

Stereotactic angiography has been the traditional database for AVM diagnosis, treatment planning and follow-up (Figs. 1 and 2). However, the advent of non-invasive MRI may change the "gold standard" of conventional angiography for AVM imaging (Figs. 3 and 4). Preliminary correlates between MRI, CT, and stereotactic angiography have been reported [4, 22, 23]. An inherent problem in stereotactic angio-

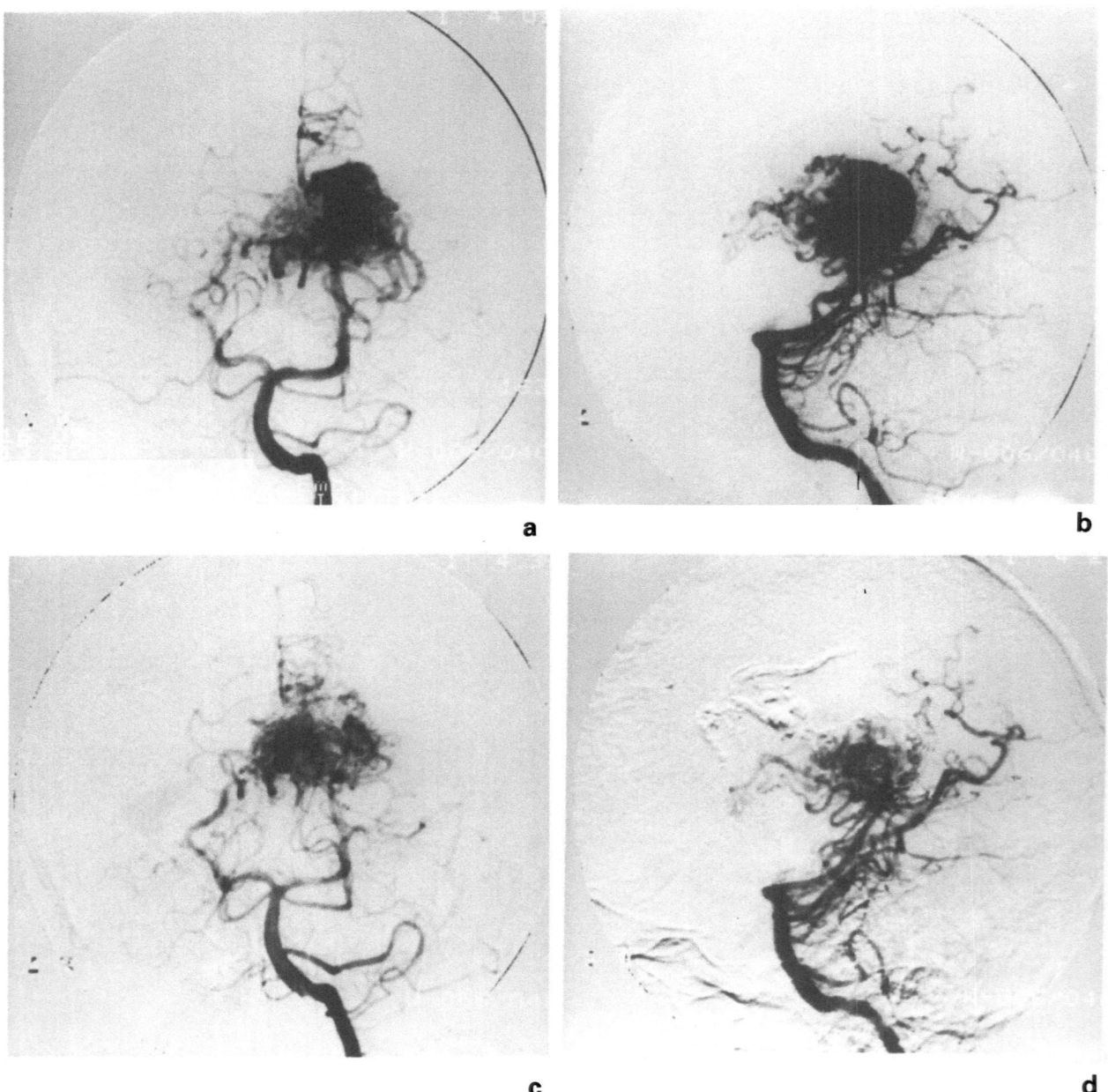

Fig. 2. (a, b) Left vertebral pre-embolization AP + lateral projection. (c, d) Left vertebral post-embolization AP + lateral

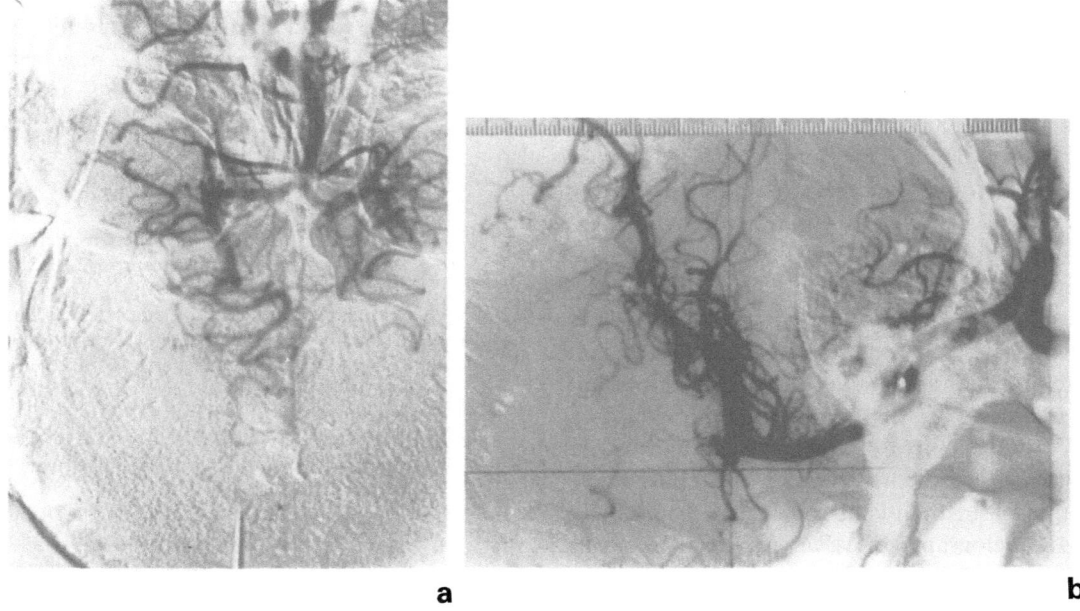

Fig. 3. Left vertebral 2 years post gamma knife (there remains some filling from ICA). (a) Antero-posterior projection. (b) Lateral projection

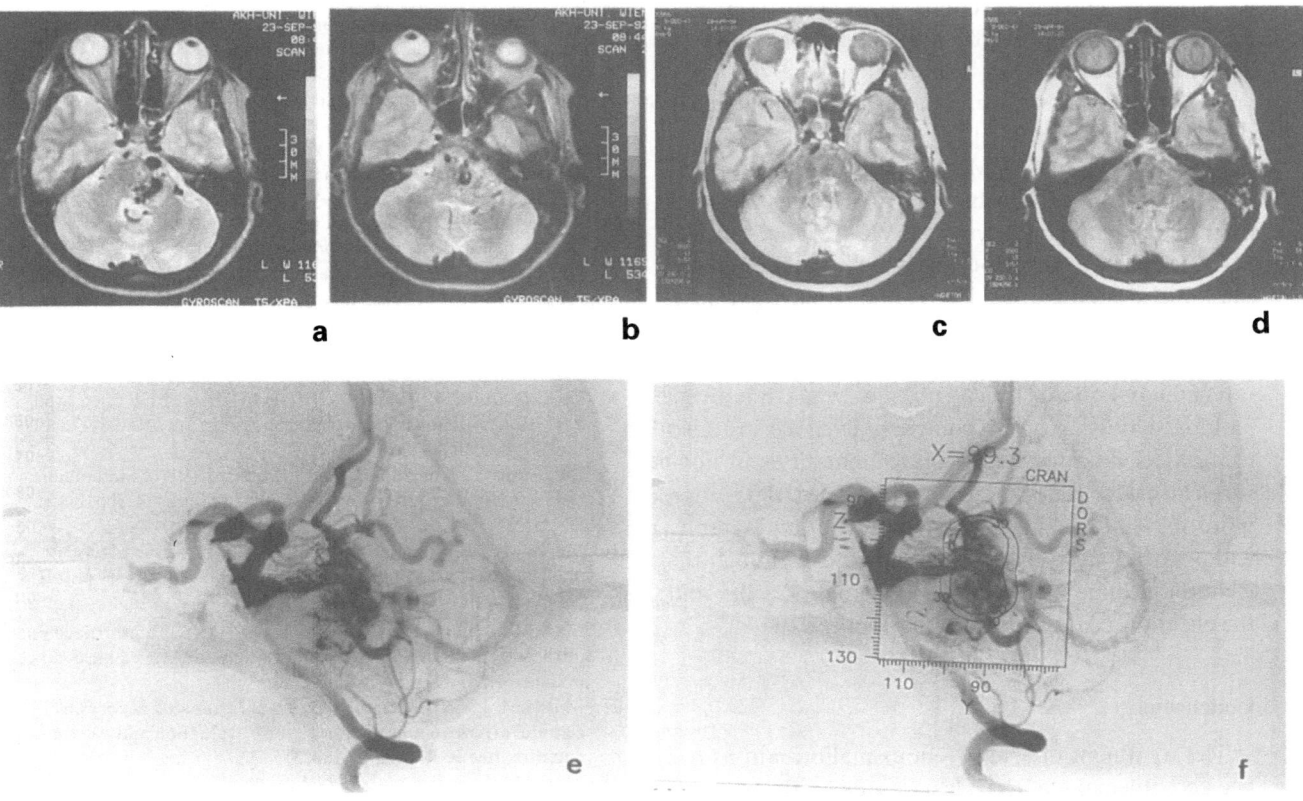

Fig. 4. (a, b) Pre-treatment MRI slices, (c, d) follow-up 18 months post gamma knife MRI. (e) Pre-treatment stereotactic angiography. (f) Same as (e) with gamma-knife plan overlay

graphy becomes magnified when dealing with an irregularly shaped AVM. The high resolution of current MRI techniques provides thin slice axial data which can allow accurate identification of nidus size, location, and shape [6, 22]. Stereotactic angiography has also been known to underestimate the size of low lying AVMs below the petrous pyramids. Further limitations of angiography have been elucidated [1]. Extensive research over the last decade has established MRI as a unique diagnostic modality for intracranial studies. Several comparisons of MRI technology to stereotactic angiography illustrate an important role of MRI currently in treatment paradigms [4, 22, 23]. Work in the area of gradient echo and bipolar flow-encoding gradient schemes has enabled the visualization of medium caliber vessels forming the basis of MR angiography or MRA [5]. Positive correllation of MRI gradient recalled echo (GRE) acquisitions with stereotactic angiography have also been performed [22, 23]. Two MRI techniques, 3D time of flight technique and 2D phase contrast angiography are compared favourably to stereotactic angiography. The 3D time of of flight technique is valuable for visualizing the AVM nidus and fastflow components. The 2D phase-contrast MRI has a shorter acquisition time and can detect slow flow AVMs. Employing these methods, only 2 of 21 AVMs were better demonstrated by stereotactic angiography [22].

The volume of an AVM, critical to treatment planning was also found to be estimated better by MRI than biplanar angiography [4]. We feel that current MRI techniques are not ready to entirely replace stereotactic angiography. For gamma knife treatment, we utilize a combined treatment protocol, gathering data from both modalities and thus insuring an accurate minimal radiosurgical margin, while not overlooking a crucial AVM compartment. We are also using MRI data for follow-up examinations in nonsurgical cases. In post-surgical cases, MRI is often quite misleading and thus stereotactic angiography will probably never be entirely replaced, although the technological advances in this imaging modality and the effect on radiosurgery are both phenomenal.

Conclusion

The treatment of arteriovenous malformations has been complemented in the last decade by the progress of radiosurgery. Radiosurgery in our institution is used primarily as an adjunct to embolization and surgery.

We have found the adverse effects minimal as has been reported in other series. MRI is now being used extensively in radiosurgical planning and follow-up with advantages in many cases over angiography.

References

1. Bova F, Friedman W (1991) Stereotactic angiography: an inadequate database for radiosurgery? Int J Radiat Oncol Biol Phys 20:891–895
2. Columbo F, Benedetti A, Pozza F (1985) External stereotactic irradiation by linear accelerator. Neurosurgery 16:154–159
3. Columbo F, Benedetti, Pozza F (1989) Linear accelerator radiosurgery of cerebral arteriovenous malformations. Neurosurgery 24:833–840
4. Frahm J, Haase A, Matthaei D (1986) Rapid NMR imaging of dynamic processes using the FLASH technique. Magn Reson Med 3:321–327
5. Guo WY, Lundquist C, Karlsson B, Kihlstrom L, Steiner L (1993) Gamma knife surgery of cerebral arteriovenous malformations: serial MR imaging studies after radiosurgery. Int J Radiat Oncol Biol Phys 25:315–323
6. Guo WY, Nordell B, Karlsson B, Soderman M, Lindquist M, Ericson K, Frank A, Lax F, Lindquist C (1993) Target delineation in radiosurgery for cerebral arteriovenous malformations. Acta Radiol 34:457–463
7. Heros R, Korosue K (1990) Radiation treatment of cerebral arteriovenous malformations. N Engl J Med 323:127–129
8. Huston J, Rufenacht D, Ehman R, Wiebers D (1991) Intracranial aneusysms and vascular malformations: comparison of time-of-flight and phase-contrast MR angiography. Radiology 181:721–3
9. Hamilton M, Spetzler R (1993) The prospective application of a grading system for arteriovenous malformations. Neurosurgery 34:2–7
10. Keller P, Drayer B, Fram E, Williams K, Domoulin C, Souza S (1989) MR angiography with two-dimensional display: work in Progress. Radiology 173:527–9
11. Kjellberg R (1983) Bragg peak proton beam therapy for arteriovenous malformations of the brain. Clin Neurosurg 31:248–268
12. Kjellberg R, Hanamura T, Davis K, Lyons S, Adams R (1983) Bragg peak proton beam therapy for arteriovenous malformations of the brain. N Engl J Med 309:269–274
13. Leksell L (1983) Steriotactic radiosurgery. J Neurol Neurosurg Psychiatry 46:797–803
14. Lo E, DeLaPaz R, Frankel K (1991) MRI and PET of delayed heavy-ion radiation injury in the rabbit brain. Int J Radiat Oncol Biol Phys 20:689–696
15. Lundsford L, Kondziolka D, Flickinger J (1991) Stereotactic radiosurgery for arteriovenous malformations of the brain. J Neurosurg 75:512–524
16. Marks M, DeLaPaz R, Fabrikant J (1988) Intracranial vascular malformations: imaging of charged-particle radiosurgery part II. complications. Radiology 168:457–462
17. Marks M, Lane B, Steinberg G, Chang P (1990) Hemorrhage in intracerebral arteriovenous malformations: angiographic determinants. Radiology 176:807–813
18. Marks M, Lane B, Steinberg G (1992) Intranidus aneurysms in cerebral arteriovenous malformations: evaluation and endovascular treatment. Radiology 183:355–360
19. Marks M, Lane B, Steinberg G, Fabrikant J, Levy R, Frankel K, Phillips M (1993) Endovascular treatment of cerebral arteriovenous malformations following radiosurgery. AJNR 14:297–303

20. McCormick W (1984) Pathology of vascular malformations of the brain. In: Wilson C, Stein B (eds) Intracranial arteriovenous malformations. Williams and Wilkins, Baltimore, pp 44–63

21. Oglivy C (1990) Radiation therapy for arteriovenous malformations: a review. Neurosurgery 26:725–735

22. Petereit D, Mehta M, Turski P, Levin A, Strother C (1993) Treatment of arteriovenous malformations with steriotactic radiosurgery employing both magnetic resonance angiography and standard angiography as a database. Int J Radiat Oncol Biol Phys 25:309–313

23. Quisling R, Peters K, Friedman W, Tart R (1991) Persistant nidus blood flow in cerebral arteriovenous malformation after stereotactic radiosurgery: MR imaging assessment. Radiology 180:785–791

24. Sisti M, Kader A, Stein B (1993) Microsurgery for 67 intracranial arteriovenous malformations less than 3 cm in diameter. J Neurosurg 79:653–660

25. Steinberg G, Fabrikant J, Marks M, Levy R, Frankel K, Phillips M, Sheur L, Silverberg G (1990) Stereotactic heavy charged particle Bragg peak radiation for intracranial arteriovenous malformations. N Eng J Med 323:96–101

26. Steiner L (1984) Treatment of arteriovenous malformations by radiosurgery. In: Wilson C, Stein B (eds) Intracranial arteriovenous malformations. Williams and Wilkins, Baltimore, pp 295–313

27. Steiner L, Leksell L, Forster D (1974) Steriotactic radiosurgery in arteriovenous malformations. Acta Neurochir (Wien) [Suppl] 21:195–209

28. Steiner L, Lindquist C, Adler J (1992) Clinical outcome of radiosurgery for cerebral arteriovenous malformations. J Neurosurg 77:1–8

29. Steiner L, Lindquist C, Steiner M (1992) Radiosurgery. Adv Tech Stand Neurosurg 19:19–102

30. Steiner L, Lindquist C, Cail W, Karlsson B, Steiner M (1993) Microsurgery and radiosurgery in brain arteriovenous malformations. J Neurosurg 79:647–652

31. Yamaguchi N, Yamashima T, Yamashita J (1991) A histopathological and flow cytometric study of dog brain endothelial cell injuries in delayed radiation necrosis. J Neurosurg 74:625–632

Correspondence: David I. Levy, Neurochirurgische Universitätsklinik, Währinger Gürtel 18–20, A-1090 Wien, Austria.

Acta Neurochir (1995) [Suppl] 63: 68–72

Treatment of Symptomatic AOVMs with Radiosurgery

Y. Kida, T. Kobayashi, and **T. Tanaka**

Department of Neurosurgery, Komaki City Hospital, Jhobusi, Komaki, Japan

Summary

In spite of great success in the treatment cerebral AVMs with stereotactic radiosurgery, the role of this treatment modality in angiographically occult vascular malformations (AOVMs) is not recognized. Since the installation of the Gamma-knife, we have treated 20 cases of AOVMs by radiosurgery. There were 13 males and 7 females, the age ranged from 3 to 58 years with an average age of 34.0 years. Their clinical presentations at the onset were haemorrhage in 11, convulsive seizure in 7 and progressive neurological deficits in 2. Two cases had multiple lesions. Among 20 symptomatic lesions, 14 were located supratentorially, 4 in the brain stem and 2 in the cerebellar hemispheres. Following localization with MRI and dose planning, the lesions were treated by radiosurgery and the doses ranged from 15 to 20 Gy at the margins. Follow-up studies indicate a significant control of rebleeding as well as of the convulsive seizure. Imaging studies demonstrated the shrinkage of the lesion in 3 and reduced enhancement with Gadolinium-DTPA in some others. Adverse effects, chiefly related to radiation-induced oedema, occurred in 5. But they were generally mild and well controlled by medication. Thus the preliminary results indicate a certain usefulness of radiosurgery in the treatment of symptomatic AOVMs.

Keywords: Arterio-venous malformation; cavernous angioma; radiosurgery; vascular malformation; venous angioma.

Introduction

The treatment method of AOVM (angiographically occult vascular malformation) or cavernoma has been controversial, partly because the natural history of this disease has not been fully clarified. Currently the cases associated with intracranial haemorrhage or with intractable seizure are suitable for operative resection or other treatment modalities. AOVMs are similar to AVMs as a pathological entity as well as in clinical presentations [4, 5]. Therefore radiosurgery might be indicated for the treatment of this disease [3]. Since the installation of the gamma-knife during May 1991 to August 1992, we have treated more than 350 cases of various intracranial lesions by radiosurgery, in which 7.2% of AOVMs are included. In this paper the early responses of this disease following radiosurgery are reported.

Materials and Methods

This Gamma-knife containing 201 Cobalt-60 sources, can deliver high doses of gamma-rays to the target volume with sharp dose gradients. After fixing the head of patient in Leksell's stereotactic frame, the localization with MRI and the dose planning with a computer system are carried out. Since T2-weighted or PD (proton density) images show the lesions of AOVM more clearly than those of plain or enhanced Tl-weighted MRI, the former are usually used for localization (Fig. 1). Four types of collimators, 4, 8, 14 and 18 mm in diameter, are utilized alone or in combination for obtaining adequate dose distributions.

There are 13 males and 7 females, with an age range from 3 to 58 years (mean 34.0). Among them 7 cases had episodes of convulsive seizures or unconscious attacks, 11 had intracranial haemorrhage, once in 5, twice in 5 and more than 3 times in 1 case (Table 1). The other 2 cases had progressive neurological deficits like hemiparesis or hemisensory disturbance. All have characteristic findings of irregular high signal intensity core with a low signal intensity rim on T2-weighted MRI. Varied enhancements with Gadolinium-DTPA were demonstrated in more than half of the lesions and were classified in terms of moderate ($++$), slight ($+$) and negative ($-$) enhancement (Fig. 2). Including 39 lesions of 20 cases, the locations were most frequent in the temporal lobe (11), followed by frontal (7), parietal (7), thalamus (3), midbrain (4), pons (4) and cerebellum (3). The mean diameters of the lesions ranged from 4.0 to 27.0 mm with an average of 12.2 mm. Maximum and marginal doses in each lesion were determined depending on the size and location. Follow-up studies with MRI were performed every 3 months, and the sizes, enhancement patterns on MRI as well as changes of the surrounding brain were carefully evaluated. Neurological changes and the episodes of rebleeding or frequency of convulsive seizures were also recorded.

Results

a) Treatment Doses of Radiosurgery

Treatment doses related to the sizes of AOVM are demonstrated in the table (Table 2). Most of the lesions

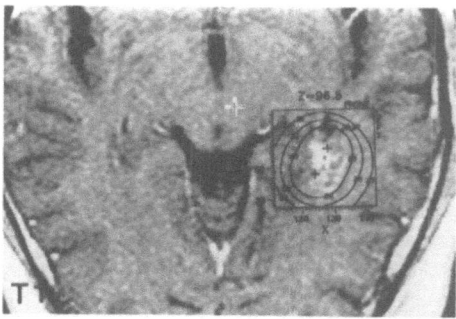

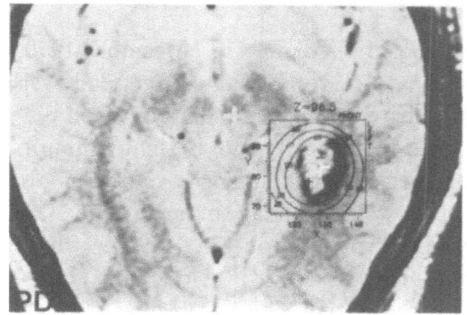

Fig. 1. AOVM (angiographically occult vascular malformation) in the left temporal lobe is clearly visualized in proton density image (lower) rather than enhanced T1-weighted MRI (upper)

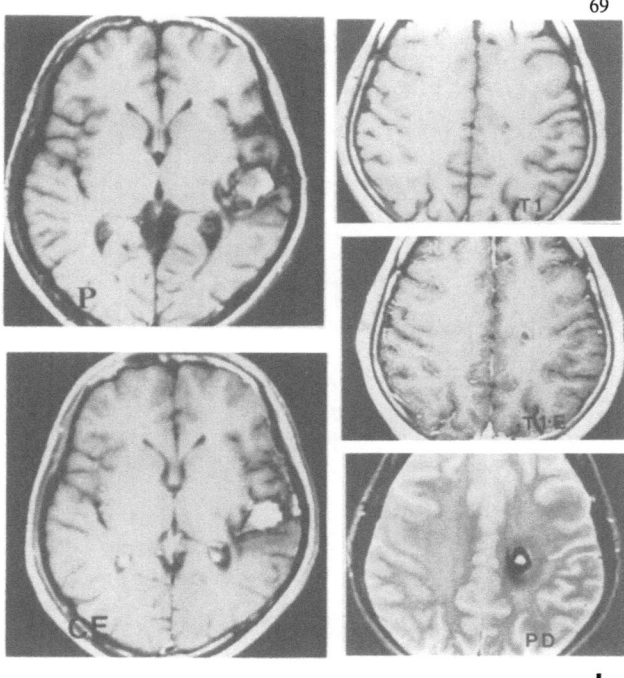

a   **b**

Fig. 2. Enhancement patterns with gadolinium-DTPA on T1-weighted MRI are varied in cases of AOVM. (a) Moderate enhancement. (b) Minor enhancement

Table 1. *Clinical Presentation of AOVM (20 Cases)*

Convulsive seizure	7
Haemorrhage	11
	once 5
	twice 5
	3 ≤ 1
Neurological deficit	2

Location of AOVM (20 Cases)

Frontal lobe	7
Temporal lobe	11
Parietal lobe	7
Thalamus	3
Midbrain	4
Pons	4
Cerebellum	3

Table 2. *Radiosurgery of AOVM (20 Cases)*

	Size of AOVM	No.	Max. dose	Marg. dose (mean)
1	10 > mm	21	25–40	15–25.2 (19.8)
2	10–15	6	36–44	18–20 (17.3)
3	15–20	8	30–44	16–22 (18.6)
4	20–25	3	28–44	14–22 (17.0)
5	25–30	1	25	11.3 (11.3)
Mean	12.2 mm	39	25–44	11.3 – 25.2 (18.7 Gy)

except for 4 are less than 20 mm in diameter, and were treated with marginal doses of almost 20 Gy. However AOVMs larger than 20 mm and those located in eloquent areas like the brain stem were usually treated with lower marginal doses. AOVMs in the brain stem were treated with 13 to 18 Gy at the margins in this series (Fig. 3). Actually 39 lesions of 20 cases received 18.7 Gy of a mean marginal dose, meanwhile the maximum doses ranged from 25 to 44 Gy.

b) Clinical Presentations

Clinically haemorrhages after radiosurgery are not recorded in any cases in the mean follow-up period of 9.9 months. Four cases still have convulsive seizures, but less frequently than before radiosurgery in 3, and rather increased in 1. Among 20 cases, 7 were clinically improved, 9 showed no change and another 4 experienced a transient deterioration due to radiation-induced oedema (Table 3).

c) Radiological Findings

MRI studies disclosed a shrinkage of the lesions in 3, in which one lesion almost disappeared. A decreased

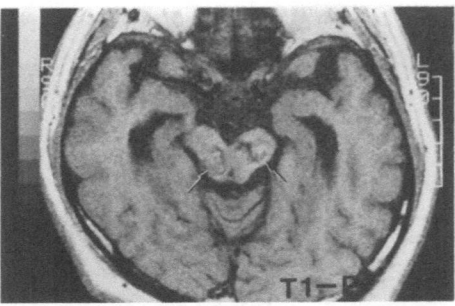
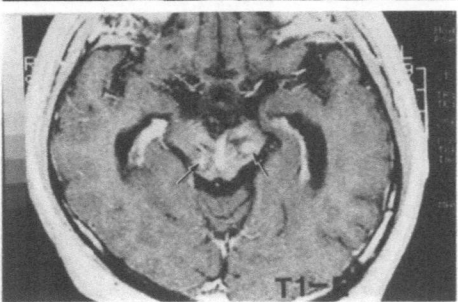

Fig. 3. Two AOVMs in the midbrain are shown (arrows). They were treated with a marginal dose of 15 Gy on the 60% isodose line. Plain (upper) and enhanced T1-weighted MRI (lower)

Table 3. *Clinical Outcome (20 Cases, Mean Follow-up 9.9 M)*

Improved		7
No Change		9
Worsened by oedema		4
Rebleeding		0
Convulsive seizure	decreased	3
	increased	1
	no seizure	16

enhancement with Gadolinium-DTPA was found in another 3 lesions. However the majority of the lesions demonstrated no obvious changes in and around the central cores. Increased oedema surrounding the lesions appeared in 6 AOVMs of 5 cases, in which 4 were symptomatic (Table 4).

d) Adverse Effects

No adverse effects were seen during and immediately after radiosurgical procedures. Radiation-induced oedema occurred in 5 cases radiologically, and 4 of them demonstrated a transient worsening of neurological signs at 3, 5, 6, 9 months later respectively.

Table 4. *Follow-up Results on MRI (20 Cases)*

Disappeared	1
Decreased in size	2
Decreased enhancement	3
No change	14
Increased oedema	5

e) Illustrative Cases

Case 1. Female, aged 58 years. On November 1990, she had an episode of rotational vertigo and was admitted to a nearby hospital. CT on admission disclosed a abnormal high density spot in right temporal lobe. MRI showed high signal intensity spot with low intensity rim on Tl-weighted image indicating AOVM. Radiosurgery was carried out on May 1991, in which the lesion measuring $8 \times 7 \times 8$ mm in diameter received 21.6 Gy at the margin. This AOVM has gradually reduced in size and finally showed complete resolution 12 months later (Fig. 4).

Case 2. Man, aged 28 years. He had an initial convulsive seizure when he was 23 years old. The second seizure occurred in May 1992. Neuro-radiological studies at the time demonstrated an AVOM in the right temporal lobe and he was referred to us for treatment by radiosurgery. The lesion, measuring $20 \times 20 \times 13$ mm in diameter, received 21 Gy at the margin using one 18 mm collimator. He has had no seizures thereafter and has been well with regard to daily activity. MRI showed a considerable decrease of AOVM 3 months later (Fig. 5).

Discussion

Angiographically occult vascular malformation (AOVM), which is defined as an angiographically negative vascular malformation may includes various clinical entities like a thrombosed AVM [1, 6], cavernous angioma or venous angioma [7–10]. Lobato *et al.* reported that of 241 AOVMs 43.8% were thrombosed AVMs, 31.2% were cavernous angiomas, 9.9% venous angiomas, 3.8% capillary telangioectases and 11% of mixed or unclassified angiomas [4]. AOVMs are found sometimes incidentally or with episodes of convulsive seizures. Although the natural history of this disease as well as the incidence of haemorrhage has not been well understood, it is generally believed that the clinical features are similar to those of AVMs (arterio-venous

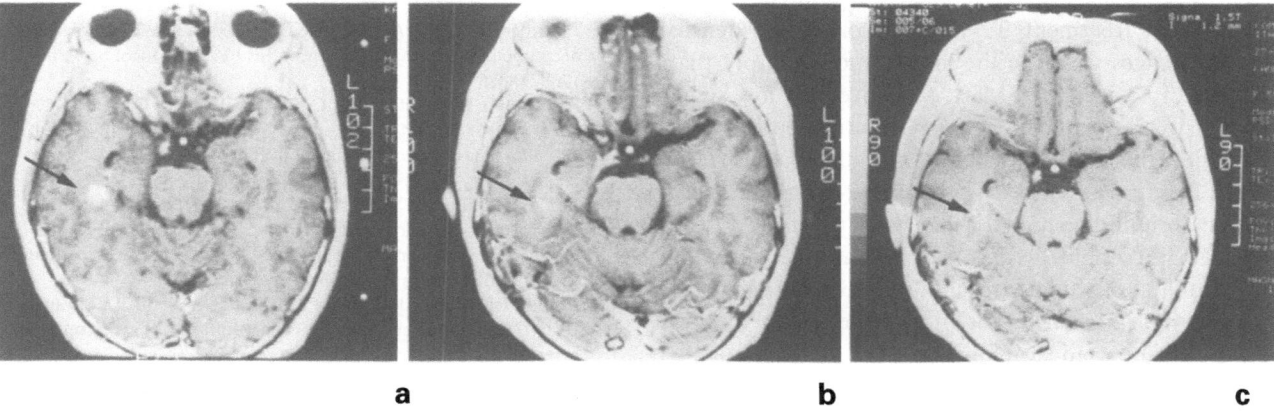

a   **b**   **c**

Fig. 4. A small AOVM in right temporal lobe demonstrated a consistent shrinkage (arrows) over 12 months after the radiosurgery with a marginal dose of 21.6 Gy. (a) 3 months, (b) 6 months, (c) 12 months

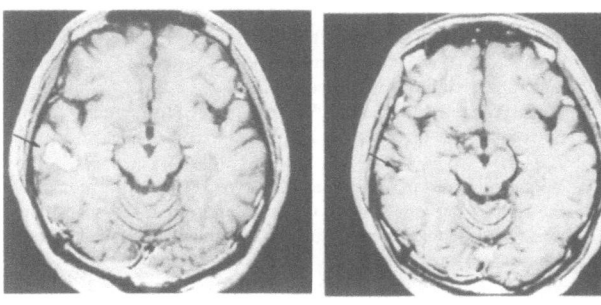

Fig. 5. AOVM in right temporal lobe disclosed a marked shrinkage (arrows) only 3 months after the radiosurgery with a marginal dose of 21 Gy on the 70% isodose line

malformation) [5]. In the series of Tagle *et al.* [9], the clinical presentations of cavernous angioma were convulsive seizure (53.5%), increased ICP (30.8%) or neurological deficits (15.8%). In contrast Lobato *et al.* [5] mentioned that the initial presentations of AOVM due to haemorrhage occurred in 61.8%, to convulsive seizure in 27.2% and to neurological deficit in 7.2%. Our own series indicate 55% were due to haemorrhage, 35% to seizure and 20% to neurological deficit, which is similar to the studies by Lobato *et al.* In comparison with AVMs, haemorrhage from AOVMs are usually more frequent and associate with higher morbidity [5]. In fact many of our cases had repeated bleeding in a relatively short period of time once the initial episode had occurred. Those symptomatic AOVMs were currently scheduled for operative interventions if they were resectable. Previous reports [4, 6, 9] emphasized that the surgical extirpation of peripherally located AOVMs is preferable since these lesions are well circumscribed. Several reports [13, 14] indicated that even the lesions in the brain stem could be successfully

resected with acceptable morbidity. It has been controversial whether this kind of disease is suitable for radiosurgery or not. Kondziolka *et al.* [3] stressed from their preliminary experience that radiosurgery by gamma-knife was useful for controlling AOVMs since almost all the cases showed no bleeding and were clinically stable, and 4 out of 24 cases demonstrated a shrinkage of the lesion after the treatment. In contrast Weil *et al.* [13] mentioned that stereotactic radiosurgery in the treatment of brain stem AOVMs was not recommended because of the lack of evidence of therapeutic benefits as well as complications related to radiation-induced injury. In our cases no bleeding from AOVMs occurred after radiosurgery, and the convulsive seizures were less frequent. On MRI some of AOVMs showed a significant shrinkage, or reduced contrast enhancement in a relatively short period of time. Of course long-term follow-up is required to see whether rebleeding or convulsive seizures can be fully controlled.

In our series the undue effects related to radiation-induced oedema [1] are usually transient and acceptable even in the cases affecting the brain stem. The treatment doses at the periphery approximated 20 Gy to the lesions in the cerebral hemisphere, and 15 Gy to brain stem cases, causing symptomatic oedema in 4 (20%). This is almost equivalent to the doses of Kondziolka *et al.* [3], in which complications occurred in 5 out of 24 cases (20.8%), but they were reportedly transient. Therefore radiosurgery seems to be useful to control AOVMs, especially when the surgical intervention is difficult or impossible.

Several other questions are raised in the radiosurgery of AOVMs. One thing is how to determine localization for treatment. T2-weighted or proton density MRI images visualize the lesions more sharply than those of T1-weighted MRI. Moreover the low signal intensity rim indicating haemosiderin deposits (and possibly there is no indication to irradiate), is not clear in T1-weighted images. Therefore T2-weighted or PD images should be used for localization. Since AOVMs are angiographically occult here is another question: What kind of studies are suitable and required for the follow-up. In our experience some of the lesions showed apparent shrinkage on MRI, but this must be carefully differentiated from the concomitant haematomas. Enhancement patterns are helpful for evaluating the effects because they may indicate the activity or permeability of the lesions. In cases presenting convulsive seizures with abnormal electroencephalograms (EEG), this electrophysiological study may be useful. The final evaluation definitely depends on the clinical course and outcome after radiosurgery. It is extremely important to see how rebleeding and convulsive seizures are subsequently controlled.

Conclusion

Preliminary experience with radiosurgery of 20 cases of AOVM is reported. Using the gamma-knife, AOVMs were treated with a mean marginal dose of 18.7 Gy. Clinical data as well as imaging studies with MRI indicate some evidence of success. Radiosurgery can be utilized for the treatment of AOVMs, especially for those lesions which are surgically inaccessible.

References

1. Ebeling JD, Tranmer BI, Davis KA, Kindt GW, DeMasters (1988) Thrombosed arteriovenous malformations: a type of occult vascular malformation. Neurosurgery 23: 605–610
2. Flickinger JC (1989) An integrated logistic formula for prediction of complications from radiosurgery. Int J Radiat Oncol Biol Phys 17: 879–885
3. Kondziolka D, Lunsford LD, Coffey RJ, Bissonett DJ, Flickinger JC (1990) Stereotactic radiosurgery of angiographically occult vascular malformations: indication and preliminary experience. Neurosurgery 6: 892–900
4. Lobato RD, Perez C, Rivas JJ, Cordobes F (1988) Clinical radiological and pathological spectrum of angiographically occult intracranial vascular malformations. Analysis of 21 cases and review of the literature. J Neurosurg 68: 518–531
5. Lobato RD, Rivas JJ, Gomez PA, Cabrena A, Sarabia R, Lamas E (1992) Comparison of the clinical presentation of symptomatic arteriovenous malformations (angiographically visualized) and occult vascular malformations. Neurosurgery 31: 391–397
6. Ogilvy CS, Heros RC, Ojemann RG, New PF, (1988) Angiographically occult arteriovenous malformations. J Neurosurg 69: 350–355
7. Rigamonti D, Drayer BP, Johnson PC, Hadley MN, Zabramski J Spetzler RF (1987) The MRI appearance of cavernous malformations (angiomas). J Neurosurg 67: 518–524
8. Simard JM, Garcia-Bengochea F, Ballinger WE, Mickle JP, Quisling RG (1986) Cavernous angioma: a review of 126 collected and 12 new clinical cases. Neurosurgery 18: 162–172
9. Tagle P, Huete I, Mendez J, Villar SD (1986) Intracranial cavernous angioma: presentation and management. J Neurosurg 64: 720–723
10. Vaquero J, Salazar J, Martinez R, Bravo G (1987) Cavernomas of the central nervous system: Clinical syndromes, CT scan diagnosis, and prognosis after surgical treatment in 25 cases. Acta Neurochir (Wien) 85: 29–33
11. Voigt S, Yasargil MG (1976) Cerebral cavernous haemangiomas or cavernomas. Incidence, pathology, localization, diagnosis clinical features and treatment. Review of the literature and report of an unusual case. Neurochirugia (Stuttg) 19: 59–68
12. Wakai S, Ueda Y, Inoh S, Nagai M (1985) Angiographically occult angiomas: a report of 13 cases with analysis of the cases documented in the literature. Neurosurgery 17: 549–556
13. Weil S, Tew JM, Steiner L (1990) Comparison of radiosurgery and microsurgery for treatment of cavernous malformations of the brain stem. J Neurosurg 72: 336A
14. Yoshimoto T, Suzuki J (1986) Radical surgery on cavernous angioma of the brain stem. Surg Neurol 26: 72–78

Correspondence: Yoshihisa Kida, M.D., Department of Neurosurgery, Komaki City Hospital, 1–20, Jhobusi, Komaki City, Aichi Pref., Japan.

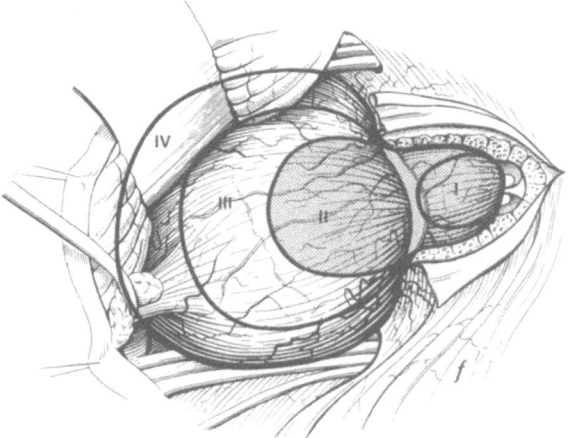

Fig. 1. Grading system for neurinomas

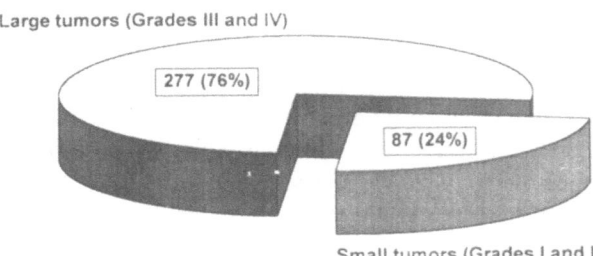

Large tumors (Grades III and IV)

277 (76%)

87 (24%)

Small tumors (Grades I and II)

Fig. 2. Acoustic neurinomas operated on between 1980 and 1993. Total number of neurinomas: 364 (100%), OP-mortality: 0.5%

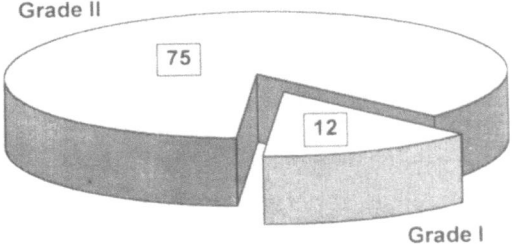

Grade II

75

12

Grade I

Fig. 3. Acoustic neurinomas–small tumours (1980–1993). Total number: 87

types of acoustic neurinomas is an important consideration for the surgeon. The surgeon can usually identify and expose the vestibulo-cochlear nerve and its main components at its origin from the brain stem, that is, the pontobulbar sulcus. The original facial nerve is located in front of CN VIII [15, 16, 32, 33].

As the CN VIII originates from the brain stem, the nerve divides into its vestibular and the cochlear branch and it may be possible to distinguish clearly the superior and inferior vestibular nerves. The relation between CN VIII and the neurinoma will be discussed later.

It is important to remember that surgical and neuroanatomical studies, particularly those of Neely and Ylikoski and others [24, 25, 44, 45], showed that in the region of the fundus of the internal

auditory meatus, the inferior vestibular nerve is implicated by tumour in more than 70% of cases, as is the superior vestibular nerve in 30% and the cochlear nerve in more than 20% of cases (Fig. 5). This study suggests that in the majority of cases acoustic neurinomas originate from the vestibular portion of the eighth cranial nerve during its intrameatal course but may also involve other components of this nerve. All of these tumours originate in the neurilemmal segment of the nerve, lateral to the glial-neurilemmal junction [15, 16].

Surgical Considerations

In all our cases the patients were operated on in the semi-sitting position. In more than 80% of cases with medium-sized and large neurinomas as well as in 100% of small neurinomas, the origin of the vestibulocochlear nerve above the pontomedullary sulcus can be located by gentle medial retraction of cerebellar hemisphere and flocculus. In larger tumours the debulked tumour has to be retracted laterally. Now the topographic relations between CN VIII and the tumour have to be carefully evaluated. Particularly in small tumours the topographic relations between CN VIII and VII are essential for the further separation of nerve and tumour.

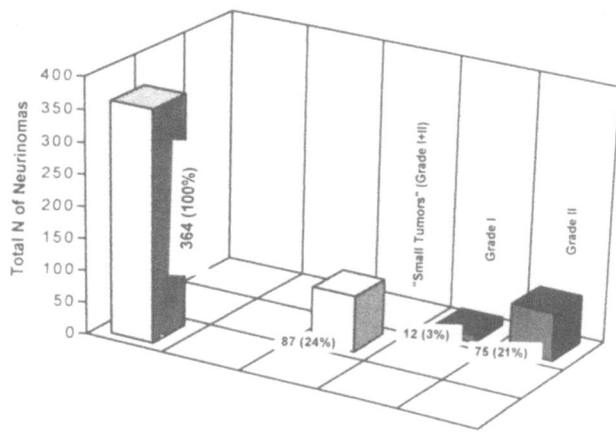

Fig. 4. Microsurgery of acoustic neurinomas operated on between 1980 and 1993 (n = 364)

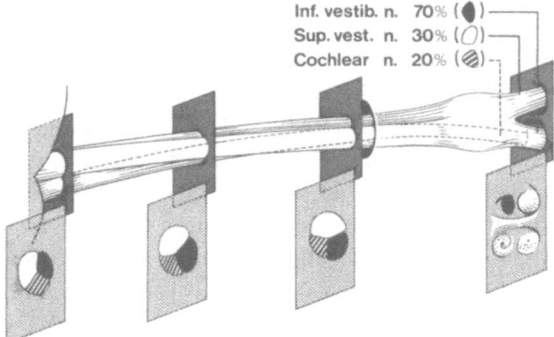

Inf. vestib. n. 70% (●)
Sup. vest. n. 30% (◐)
Cochlear n. 20% (◉)

Fig. 5.

Acta Neurochir (1995) [Suppl] 63: 73–80

Microsurgery Versus Radiosurgery in the Treatment of Small Acoustic Neurinomas

W. T. Koos, Ch. Matula, D. Levy, and **K. Kitz**

Department of Neurosurgery, University of Vienna Medical School, Wien, Austria

Summary

Microsurgical preservation of the facial nerve during removal of acoustic neurinomas can hardly be compared with microsurgery of the eighth cranial nerve. Many more anatomical and pathogenetic factors are involved that need careful consideration. In small neurinomas, of grades I and II, total extirpation of the tumour with preservation of both the facial nerve and segments of the vestibulocochlear nerve not directly involved by the tumour has become a safe and practical technique. In small acoustic neurinomas immediate facial nerve function could be preserved in 88% and "useful hearing" could be preserved in 78%. A number of different types of tumour-cranial nerve relationships could be established in small acoustic neurinomas, showing also the effects of adjusted surgical techniques on the preservation of hearing. Optimal selective separation of cranial nerves from the tumour is only possible through open surgical intervention, while radiosurgery requires the irradiation of the entire tumour/nerve complex.

Keywords: Small acoustic neurinomas; hearing; preservation; radiosurgery.

Introduction

The main aim of modern microneurosurgery of acoustic neurinomas is to achieve total tumour removal while keeping the mortality rate low and the morbidity rate within acceptable limits. Our overall operative mortality in 364 patients operated on in our department between 1980 and 1993 amounts to 2 deaths, i.e. a rate of below 0.5%. A further aim is to preserve the function of the facial and the vestibulocochlear nerves and to prevent tumour recurrence.

Advances in diagnostic and microsurgical techniques have contributed significantly to a reduction of postoperative morbidity in surgically treated acoustic neurinomas, especially in preserving facial nerve function and preserving or even improving the function of the cochlear nerve.

In small, i.e., grade I and II, acoustic neurinomas surgery can now be done under optimal conditions. Total extirpation of the tumour with preservation of both the facial nerve and segments of the vestibulocochlear nerve not directly involved has become a safe and practicable technique [2–6, 9, 11–13, 15–17, 23–25, 27–43].

Material

If function of the facial nerve as well as the vestibulo-cochlear nerve is to be preserved, tumour size and topographic variations between neurinoma and CN VII and CN VIII need to be known. We studied these criteria during microsurgical dissection of 364 neurinomas.

Grading

For the classification of tumour sizes, a grading system (grades I to IV) was introduced, using criteria from pre- and postoperative clinical, radiological (CT scan), MRI, and intra-operative observations, including surgical photographs in all cases as well as anatomical investigations [15–17]. Out of 364 acoustic neurinomas operated on by microsurgical techniques, 24% were found to be grades I and II ("small tumours"), 76% were classified grades III and IV ("large tumours") (Figs. 1–4).

Topography of the CN VIII

Microsurgical preservation of the facial nerve during removal of acoustic neurinomas can hardly be compard with the micro-surgical preservation of the eighth cranial nerve. Many more anatomical and pathogenetic factors are involved that need careful consideration. The site for identifying the 7th and 8th cranial nerves in different

Results

Preservation of Facial Nerve Function (CN VII)

Many authors have discussed the anatomical and topographic criteria which must be considered for the preservation of the function of the facial nerve [15, 16]. These criteria apply in particular for grades III and IV neurinomas. Figures 6, 7 and 8 indicate that in our series of acoustic neurinomas the CN VII cannot always be located nor preserved as an anatomical struc-

ture, a phenomenon that is encountered very rarely only (2%) with small tumours. Figures 9 and 10 graphically represent the preservation of facial nerve function in "small tumours" and "large tumours"; modern operating techniques often allow the preservation of full nerve function. Figure 11 shows the postoperative recovery of facial nerve function up to 12 and

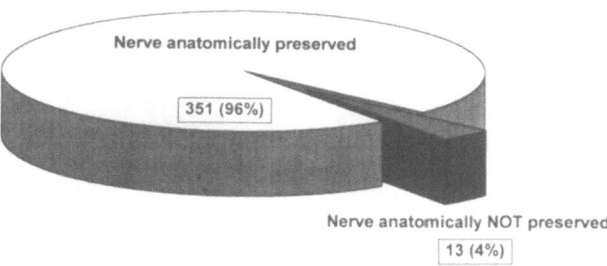

Fig. 6. Preservation of facial nerve funciton in neurinomas grades I to IV (all sizes). Postoperative results. Total number of tumours: 364

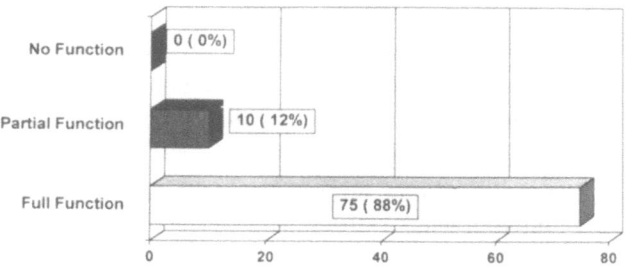

Fig. 9. Preservation of facial nerve function in neurinomas grades I and II ("small tumours"). Function of anatomically preserved nerve

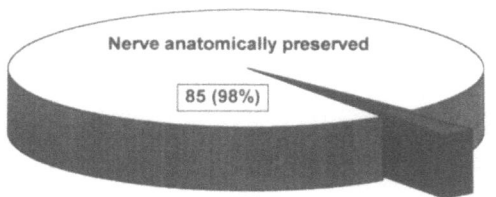

Fig. 7. Preservation of facial nerve function in neurinomas grades I and II ("small tumours"). Postoperative results. Total number of tumours: 87

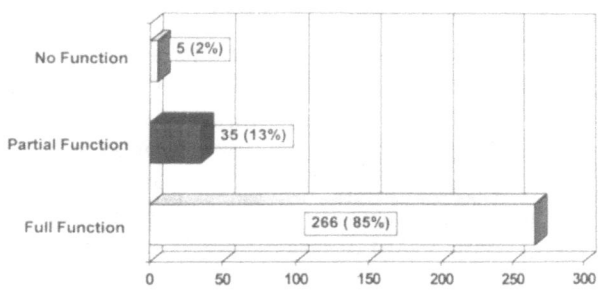

Fig. 10. Preservation of facial nerve function in neurinomas grades III and IV ("Large tumours"). Function of anatomically preserved nerve

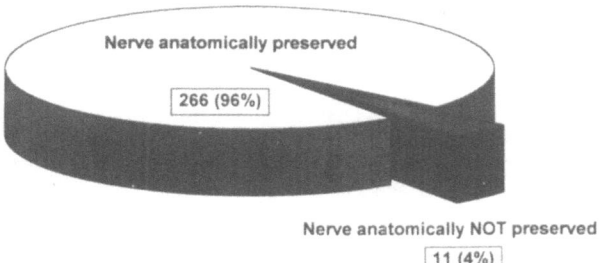

Fig. 8. Preservation of facial nerve function in neurinomas grades III and IV ("large tumours"). Postoperative results. Total number of tumours: 277

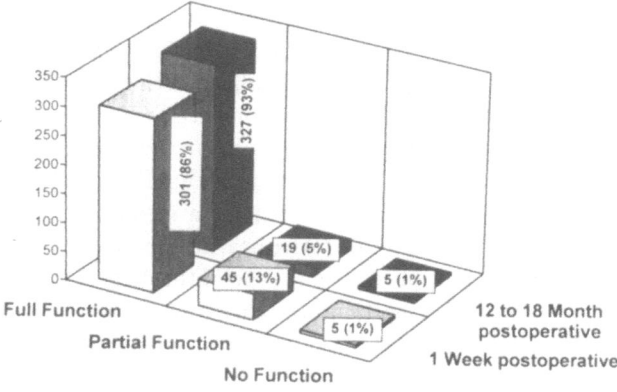

Fig. 11. Preservation of facial nervefunction in neurinomas grades I to IV ("all sizes"). One week postoperative and 12 to 18 month postoperative

18 months. Recovery to full function within 12 to 18 months after extirpation of an acoustic neurinoma is considered a good surgical result.

Preservation of Cochlear Nerve Function (CN VIII)

Prerequisites for the preservation of cochlear nerve function in acoustic neurinomas are:

1. Anatomical continuity;
2. No direct mechanical manipulation;
3. Intact arteries supplying the nerve and inner ear;
4. Adequate pre-operative cochlear function;
5. Intact inner ear (semicircular canals);
6. No extensive tumour-infiltration of nerve.

The above criteria, important for preserving cochlear funtction when extirpating acoustic neurinomas, relate to the origin of the tumour and its direction of spread. Equally important and relevant to these criteria are the shape, location, and course of the other eighth nerve components. In our experience, preservation of pre-operatively intact cochlear function definitely does not depend on tumour size alone. Our experience is in line with that of other surgeons who consider adequate pre-operative cochlear function to be a major determinant of postoperative hearing.

According to Brackman, pre-operative hearing should not be less than 50–80 dB and 80% for speech discrimination, which is considered "useful hearing" [2, 14]. With regard to surgical dissection and preservation of the cochlear nerve during total extirpation of acoustic neurinomas, Yasargil and colleagues and other authors have found that in some cases residual postoperative hearing disappears within days after surgery [43]. This phenomenon can be caused by ischaemic infarction of the cochlear nerve following intraoperative damage or postoperative vasospasm of small supplying vessels. Another possible explanation is oedema of the nerve with microhaemorrhages within the nerve. It seems of great importance that in a considerable number of patients not only the pre-operative level of function of the cochlear nerve could be preserved, but we were able to recognize a significant improvement in the postoperative hearing function [9, 27, 35]. Figure 12 represents a survey of the preservation of hearing following tumour extirpation in all of our 364 patients. Pre-operative and post-operative function of the CN VIII is compared for neurinomas of "all sizes" and this is separately shown for the categories "large tumours" and "small tumours". Figures 13 and 14 shows the extent to which hearing could be pre-

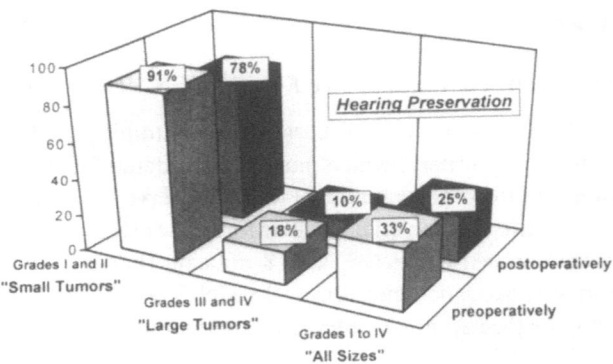

Fig. 12. Microsurgery of acoustic neurinomas operated on between 1980 and 1993. n = 364

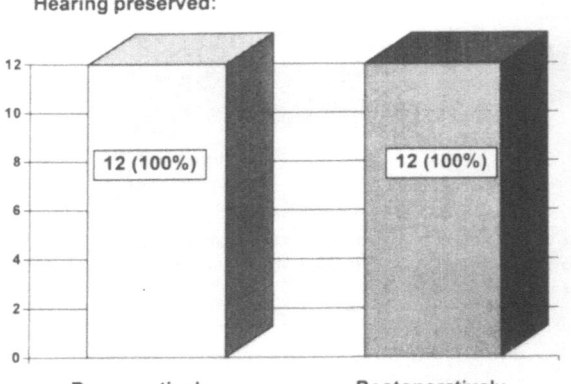

Fig. 13. Preservation of cochlear nerve function in neurinomas grade I ("small tumours"). n = 12

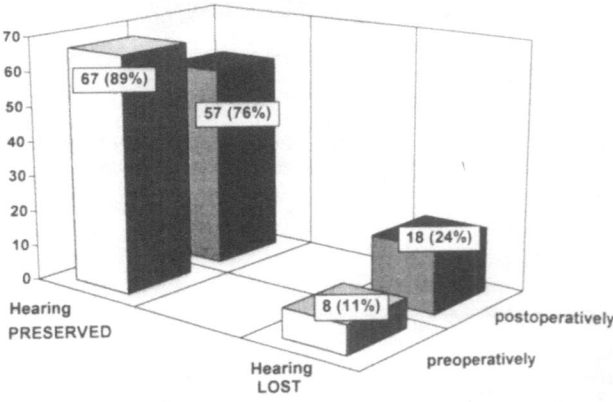

Fig. 14. Preservation of cochlear nerve function in neurinomas grade II ("small tumours"). n = 75

served in cases of small neurinomas. Special mention should be made of the excellent results achieved for grade II neurinomas, in which 100% of hearing was preserved in all 12 patients in this group.

Table 1. *Topographic Relations Between Neurinoma and CN VII and CN VIII in Cases of Small Acoustic Neurinomas (Grade II/n = 75)*

			n	%	n	%
Type	1 A	indentation of CN VIII occipitally	21	28		
Type	1 B	indentation of CN VIII from above	23	31	44	59
Type	2 A	separation between CN VIII and CN VII	13	17		
Type	2 B	separation between vestibular sections of CN VIII	11	15	24	32
Type	3	other relations of CN bundles VIII and CN VII	7	10	7	10
Total			75	100	75	100

Special Remarks About Topographic Relations Between Acoustic Neurinomas and CN VII and VIII in Cases of Small Acoustic Neurinomas (Relation Types)

A study correlating the topographic relations between acoustic neurinomas and CN VII and VIII with pre-operative and post-operative preservation of hear-ing in cases of small acoustic neurinomas turned out to yield insights of particular importance. For all of these cases, a detailed photographic documentation of the surgical intervention was available. The authors could establish three types of tumour-nerve relationships, shown in Table 1. The "types" referred to are illus-trated (Figs. 15 and 16) on the basis of surgical sketches

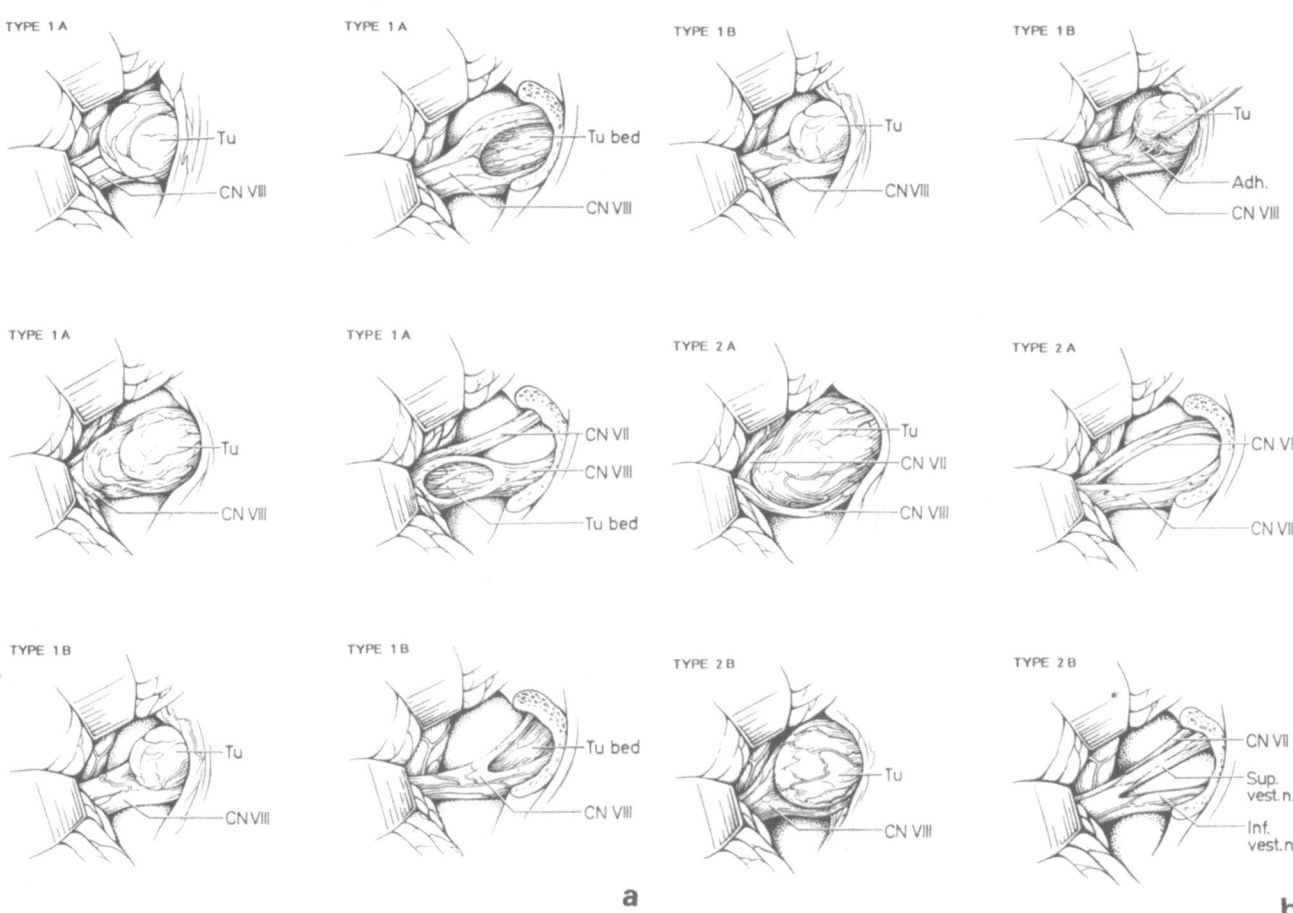

a   b

Fig. 15 a, b. (c See p. 78)

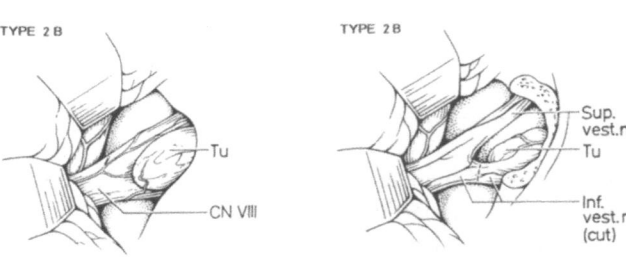

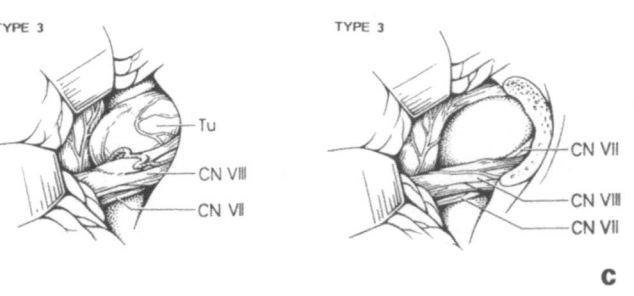

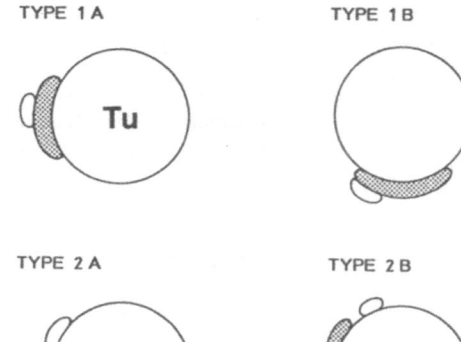

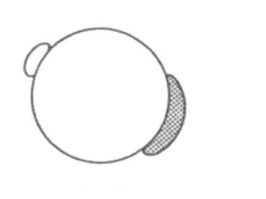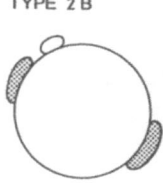

Fig. 16. Positions of cranial nerves VII and VIII with respect to neurinoma type

Fig. 15c

of nine cases of grade II acoustic neurinomas. In the majority of the cases we found a slight CN VIII depression from behind or from above; with this tumour group we succeeded in preserving hearing in the majority of cases. The same observations were made for type

2 B tumours (Table 2). Figure 14 shows the results of the surgical interventions.

Radiosurgery of Acoustic Neurinomas

Unlike open surgery, the aim of radiosurgery for acoustic neurinomas is not to remove tumour tissue but to arrest further growth. The effects of irradiation take time to develop and the result of treatment becomes difficult to assess on neuro-imaging. The follow-up time is therefore necessarily long and only during the past two years has it been possible to analyze the

Table 2. *Pre- and Postoperative Cochlear Nerve Function in Neurinomas Grade II ("Small Tumours"/n = 75) According To Relation Types of Topographic*

Preoperative hearing			Postoperative hearing		
Type	n of pt	Hearing loss	Type	n of pt	Hearing loss
1 A	21	1	1 A	20	1
1 B	23	4	1 A	19	3
2 A	13	2	2 A	11	2
2 B	11	0	2 B	11	1
3	7	1	3	6	3
	75	8 (= 11%)		67	10 (= 15%)

Total preservation of CN VIII function in 57 patients (= 76% out of 75 pt).

Table 3. *Tumour Volume and Dose Distribution of 24 Acoustic Neurinomas Treated by the Gamma Knife*

Treatment	Patient	Tumour volume (cm^3)		Maximal treatment dose (Gy)		Marginal treatment dose (Gy)		Marginal treatment isodose (Gy)	
	n	mean	range	mean	range	mean	range	mean	range
Gamma knife Surgery +	11	4.1 ± 4.2	(0.3–14.0)	25 ± 4	(15–30)	12 ± 1	(11–15)	52 ± 15	(39–93)
Gamma knife	13	4.5 ± 3.9	(0.3–15.0)	25 ± 5	(15–34)	13 ± 2	(10–17)	51 ± 10	(40–83)
Total	24	4.3 ± 4.0	(0.3–15.0)	25 ± 5	(15–34)	13 ± 2	(10–17)	51 ± 12	(39–93)

patient data critically with respect to tumour control rates and treatment complications. All experienced authors [10, 18, 20, 21, 22, 26] report transient facial neuropathy in 16 to 29% of patients as a late complication but all patients recovered function within months. Trigeminal nerve dysfunction occured in 20–33% and unlike facial neuropathy, was less likely to disappear if the initial symptoms and signs were severe. Useful hearing was preserved in 35–40% of patients 2 years after treatment [14, 18, 26]. There was no report of death or infection. Tables 3 and 4 show tumour volume and dose distribution of 24 acoustic neurinomas treated by the gamma knife. These tables show that the gamma knife may be used for primary treatment but also for a combination of open surgery and subsequent gamma knife treatment. The period of two years is too short to report late complications. At our hospital, the majority of patients have been treated by open surgery (more than 500 since 1970); radiosurgery is used in special cases only, since our results in the treatment of small acoustic neurinomas (grades I and II), as shown above, has been good.

Conclusions

The main aim of modern microneurosurgery is to achieve total tumour removal while keeping the mor-

Table 4. *Age and Sex of 24 Patients Treated for Acoustic Neurinomas by the Gamma Knife*

	Patients n	Sex m/f
Acoustic neurinomas	24	5/19
	Age (years)	
	mean 64 ± 13	range (33–84)

tality rate low and the morbidity rate within acceptable limits. Our overall operative mortality in 364 cases is 0.5%. A further aim is to preserve the function of the facial and the vestibulo-cochlear nerves and to prevent tumour recurrence.

Surgical results can be expected to be excellent if the tumour is small (grades I and II). In medium and large-sized tumours (grades III and IV) total excision should always be performed whenever circumstances allow. This yields an encouragingly high percentage of cases retaining facial nerve function (93%) and a reasonable percentage of patients with preservation (25%) of hearing. The development and utilization of special operation techniques for small acoustic neurinomas has rendered good results and has allowed preservation of CN VII and VIII function to a large extent. With specially selected acoustic neurinomas, radiosurgery constitutes an excellent supplementary treatment to open surgery; in extra-ordinary cases radiosurgery alone will be used as the sole form of treatment.

References

1. Belal A Jr, Linthicum FH Jr, House WF (1982) Acoustic tumour surgery with preservation of hearing. A histopathologic report. Am J Otol 4: 9–16
2. Brackman DE (1980) Acoustic neuroma surgery: otologic medical group results. In: Silverstein H, Norrell H (eds) Neurological surgery of the ear, Vol 2. Aesculapius, Birmingham, pp 248–259
3. Bremond G, Garcin M, Magnan J (1980) Preservation of hearing in the removal of acoustic neuroma. ("Minima" posterior approach by retrosigmoid route). J Laryngol Otol 94: 1199–1204
4. Buchheit WA, Gastaldo JA (1977) the posterior fossa approach the acoustic tumours: preservation of hearing. In: Silverstein H, Norrell H (eds) Neurological surgery of the ear, Vol 1. Aesculapius, Birmingham, pp 263–266
5. Cohen NL (1979) Acoustic neurinoma surgery with emphasis on preservation of hearing. Laryngoscope 89: 886–896
6. Cohen NL, Ransohoff J (1981) Preservation of hearing in acoustic neurinoma surgery. In: Samii M, Hanetta PJ (eds) The cranial nerves. Springer, Berlin Heidelberg New York, pp 561–568
7. Delaney G, Matheson J, Smee R (1992) Stereotactic radiosurgery: an alternative approach to the management of acoustic neuromas (letter). Med J Aust 156: 440

8. Eckermeier L, Pirsig W, Mueller D (1979) Histopathology of 30 non-operated acoustic schwannomas. Arch Otohinolaryngol 222: 1–9

9. Fischer G, Costantini JL, Marcier P (1980) Improvement of hearing after microsurgical removal of acoustic neurinomas. Neurosurgery 7: 154–159

10. Flickinger JC, Lunsford LD, Linskey ME, Duma CM, Kondziolka D (1993) Gamma knife radiosurgery for acoustic tumours: multivariate analysis of four year results. Radiother Oncol 27: 91–98

11. Glasscock ME III, Dickins JRE, Wiet RJ (1980) Preservation of hearing in acoustic tumour surgery: middle fossa technique. In: Silverstein H, Norell H (eds) Neurological surgery of the ear, Vol 2. Aesculapius, Birmingham, pp 284–286

12. Glasscock ME III, Hays JW, Miller GW, et al (1978) Preservation of hearing in tumours of the internal auditory canal and cerebellopontine angle. Laryngoscope 88: 43–55

13. Harner SG, Laws ER Jr (1981) Posterior fossa approach for removal of acoustic neurinomas. Recent experience. Arch Otolaryngol 107: 590–593

14. Kondziolka D, Lunsford LD (1993) Preservation of hearing in acoustic neurinoma surgery (letter). J Neurosurg 78: 154–156

15. Koos WT, Spetzler RF, Lang J (1993) Color atlas of microneurosurgery, 2nd Ed. Thieme, Stuttgart, Thieme and Stratton, New York

16. Koos WT, Perneczky A (1985) Suboccipital approach to acoustic neurinomas with emphasis on preservation of facial nerve and cochlear nerve function. In: Rand RW (ed) Microneurosurgery, 3rd Ed. Mosby, St. Louis pp 335–365

17. Koos WT (1988) Criteria for preservation of vestibulocochlear nerve function during microsurgical removal of acoustic neurinomas. Acta Neurochir (Wien) 92: 55–66

18. Linskey ME, Flickinger JC, Lunsford LD (1993) Cranial nerve length predicts the risk of delayed facial and trigeminal neuropathies after acoustic tumours stereotactic radiosurgery. Int J Radiat Oncol Biol Phys 25: 227–233

19. Linskey ME, Lunsford LD, Flickinger JC, Kondziolka D (1992) Stereotactic radiosurgery for acoustic tumours. Neurosurg Clin North Am 3: 191–205

20. Linskey ME, Lunsford LD, Flickinger JC (1991) Neuroimaging of acoustic nerve sheath tumours after stereotaxic radiosurgery. AJNR Am J Neuroradiol 12: 1165–1175

21. Lunsford LD, Linskey ME (1992) Stereotactic radiosurgery in the treatment of patients with acoustic tumours. Otolaryngol Clin North Am 25: 471–491

22. Lunsford LD, Kondziolka D, Flickinger JC (1992) Radiosurgery as an alternative to microsurgery of acoustic tumours. Clin Neurosurg 38: 619–634

23. MacCarty CS (1975) Acoustic neuroma and the suboccipital approach (1967–1972). Mayo Clin Proc 50: 15–16

24. Neely JG (1976) Gross and microscopic anatomy of the eighth cranial nerve in relationsip to the solitary schwannoma. Laryngoscope 91: 1512–1531

25. Neely JG, Britton BH, Greenberg SD (1976) Microscopic characteristics of the acoustic tumour in relationship to its nerve of origin. Laryngoscope 86: 984–991

26. Noren G, Greitz D, Hirsch A, Lax I (1993) Gamma knifesurgery in acoustic tumours. Acta Neurochir (Wien) Suppl 58: 104–107

27. Ojemann RG (1980) Comments on Fischer G, Constantini JL, Mercier P (1980) Improvement of hearing after microsurgical removal of acoustic neurinoma. Neurosurgery 7: 154–159

28. Ojemann RG (1978) Microsurgical suboccipital approach to cerebellopontine angel tumours. Clin Neurosurg 25: 461–479

29. Ojemann RG, Corwell RC (1978) Acoustic neuromas treated by microsurgical suboccipital operations. Prog Neurol Surg 9: 337–373

30. Piffko P, Pasztor E (1981) Operated bilateral acoustic neurinoma with preservation of hearing and facial nerve function. J Otorhinolaryngol 43: 255–261

31. Rand RW, Kurze T (1968) Preservation of vestibular, cochlear and facial nerves during microsurgical removal of acoustic tumours: report of two cases. J Neurosurg 28: 158–161

32. Rhoton AL Jr (1976) Microsurgical removal of acoustic neuromas. Surg Neurol 6: 211–219

33. Rhoton AL Jr (1985) Microsurgical anatomy of the internal acoustic meatus and facial nerve. In: Rand RW (ed) Microneurosurgery, 3rd Ed. Mosby, St Louis pp 217–235

34. Samii M (1979) Operative treatment of cerebellopontine angle tumors with special consideration of the facial and the acoustic nerve. In: Marguth F et al (eds) Advances in neurosurgery, Vol 7. Springer, Berlin Heidelberg New York pp 138–145

35. Samii M, Ohlemutz A (1981) Preservation of eighth cranial nerve in cerebello-pontine angle tumours. In: Samii M, Janetta PJ (eds) The cranial nerves. Springer, Berlin Heidelberg New York, pp 586–590

36. Smith MFW, Clancy TP, Lang JS (1977) Conservation of hearing in acoustic neurilemmoma excision. Trans Am Acad Ophthalmol Otolaryngol 84: 704–709

37. Sterkers JM (1980) Removal of bilateral and unilateral acoustic tumours with preservation of hearing: a comparison of the retrosigmoid and translabyrinthine approach. In: Silverstein H, Norrell H (eds) Neurological surgery of the ear, Vol 2. Aesculapius, Birmingham, pp 269–277

38. Sterkers JM (1979) neurinomas de l'acoustique et autres tumeurs de l'angle et du conduit auditif interne. Resultats operatoires et choix de la voie d'abord (126 cas). Ann Otolaryngol Chir Cervico fac 96: 373–386

39. Sterkers JM, Hamann KF (1979) the retrosigmoidal approach – a possibility to preserve hearing function in operations of acoustic neuromas. Arch Otorhinolaryngol 223: 463–465

40. Sterkers JM (1981) Retro-sigmoid approach for preservation of hearing in early acoustic neuroma surgery. In: Samii M, Janetta PJ (eds) The cranial nerves. Springer, Berlin Heidelberg New York, pp 586–590

41. Thomsen J, Tos M (1993) Management of acoustic neuromas. Ann Otolaryngol Chir Cervicofac 110: 179–191

42. Wanxing C (1981) Preservation of facial and acoustic nerves in total removal of large and small acoustic tumours. Report of two cases. J Neurosurg 54: 268–272

43. Yasargil MG, Smith RD, Gasser JC (1977) Microsurgical approach to acoustic neurinomas. In: Krayenbühl H (ed) Advances and technical standards in neurosurgery, Vol 4. Springer, Wien New York, pp 93–129

44. Ylikoski J, Palva T, Collan Y (1978) Eighth nerve in acoustic neuromas. Arch Otolaryngol 104: 532–537

45. Ylikoski J et al (1978) Cochlear nerve in neurilemomas. Arch Otolaryngol 104: 679–684

Correspondence: Wolfgang T. Koos, M. D., Neurochirurgische Universitätsklinik, Währinger Gürtel 18–20, A-1090 Wien, Austria.

Acta Neurochir (1995) [Suppl] 63: 81–84

The Need for Adjunctive Focused Radiation Therapy in Pituitary Adenomas

E. Knosp, A. Perneczky, K. Kitz, P. Grunert, and **A. Wild**

Department of Neurosurgery, University Clinic, Mainz, Federal Republic of Germany and Department of Neurosurgery, University Clinic, Wien, Austria

Summary

In pituitary adenomas radiation therapy regardless of the technique should be limited to surgical failures. The delayed onset of beneficial effects and the high rate of pituitary insufficiency have to be weighed against the good sugical and/or medical results in the treatment of these tumours. Unfortunately surgical outcome is almost invariably correlated with invasive growth. Invasiveness is statistically significantly correlated with tumour size, as well as with high proliferation rates, which can be measured by immunhistological methods such as mAB KI-67.

Owing to the good results of medical treatment, radiation theray is usually unnecessary in prolactinomas. Patients with persistent hypersecretion of growth hormone after unsuccessful surgery may represent the ideal candidates for radiation therapy, whereas patients with persistent Cushing's disease need cure for hypercortisolism without delay. In patients with residual tumour due to non functioning adenomas, radiation therapy should only be given if the proliferation rate is high.

Keywords: Pituitary adenoma; microsurgery; radiation therapy.

Introduction

Pituitrary adenomas are a very fascinating group of endocrine tumours, which behave differently in various terms: in their clinical appeerance, in their size, in their biological behaviour as well as in their options of treatment. Medical treatment represents the first choice of treatment in prolactinomas and allowes for disease control in the majority of patients [35, 39]. Recently medical treatment became available also for acromegaly, but with less effect on tumour shrinkage [3, 18, 29]. Surgery still is the first choice of treatment in acromegalic patients – with or without medical pretreatment – in patients with Cushing's disease and in patient with hormonal inactive adenomas. With the good results of medical and surgical treatment or in their combination, radiotherapy has no place as the first choice of treatment, mainly due to side effects and the delayed onset of benefits.

In surgical failures or in invasive growing adenomas, adjunctive radiation therapy is needed for disease control. The question however remains which modality of radiation is most effective with the least side effects [26]. With the ongoing proliferation of stereotactically focused radiation units the indication for treatment remains debateble [5, 8, 27, 31]. In the following we want to discuss the reasons for unfavourable surgical outcome in pituitary adenomas and the indications for the need of adjunctive therapy.

Methods

Factors Which Influence Surgical Cure Rates

The common denominator in unfavourable outcome in our opinion is invasiveness–regardless of the pitfalls with adenomas of different hormonal types. There is abundant evidence to suggest, that invasiveness results in a fall of cure rates as well as an increase in recurrences and/or residual tumour [2, 9, 13, 20, 21, 41].

Invasiveness can be observed macroscopically during surgery [28, 32, 33], but can also be diagnosed radiologically in plain x-ray films, CT and MRI. The radiological evidence of invasion resulted in a generally accepted classification of pituitary adenomas [12, 41]. With CT the interest has been focused on bony changes in the floor of the sella. With MRI evidence of extension or invasion into the space of the cavernous sinus became readily visible and in detail. We have tried to classify paraseller extension in using MRI criteria, and could demonstrate that surgically observed invasion was present, if the adenoma reached the lateral aspect of the intracavernous internal carotid artery [17]. Histological investigation is the most precise method available to prove invasiveness. The most common – and routinely performed tissue for histological investigation is the dura of the sellar floor, overlying the adenoma [15, 16, 20, 32, 33]. However invasion of normal pituitary gland has also been demonstrated [41]. In roughly half of reported cases (40% Selman, 51% Landolt 1987, 48% Knosp 1991) invasiveness was observed surgically, whereas in 2/3 of these cases invasiveness could be demonstrated histologically (85% Selman and 65% Landolt, 65% Knosp).

Invasiveness is Correlated to Tumour Size

Selman demonstrated, that histologically proven invasion of the sella floor is related to tumour size and was present in 85% of tumours with suprasellar extension as compared to 69% of microadenomas [33]. Unfavourable outcome has also been correlated with the high serum levels of hypersecreted hormones [1, 4]. Acromegalic patients with levels greater than 40 µg/ml [31, 40] or greater than 70 µg/ml [2] did less well than those below these levels. The same was true with prolactin levels of > 200 µg/ml [13]. Hormonal excess parallels, in general, the size of the tumour [12, 23].

Invasiveness Correlated to Growth Rates

Invasiveness has been related to aggressive and rapid growth, even when histological methods fail to demonstrate signs of malignacy. With the application of proliferation markers such as mAb Ki-67 or PCNA, growth rates can be estimated more precisely; These results clearly demonstrate, that invasive adenomas have higher growth rates [15, 16, 20]. The complication rate of trans-sphenoidal surgery for pituitary adenomas is very low; with a mortality of 0.5–2% [24]; meningitis of 1% [24], CSF leak in 2% of cases [24].

Discussion

Prolactin Secreting Adenomas

Primary treament for microprolactinomas is usually medical treatment with dopaminergic [39]. In case of drug intolerance – which occurs in about 10–15% surgical intervention is indicated. After pretreatment the shape of the tumour becomes irregular and less clearly defined by MRI, and the surgeon is often confronted with fibrotic changes and less clear tumour margins. These facts seem to adversely influence the cure rate. Conventional radiation therapy is not indicated, because of the benign course of the disease and the high risk of pituitary insufficiency in predominantly young patients [7, 34]. Focused radiation therapy therefore also lacks the clear margins necessary to define the target. It also does not yet have a clearly defined risk for pituitary insufficiency. [5, 37] although it seems to be lower than in conventional radiation therapy.

Macroprolactinomas

Usually these are large and irregularly shaped tumours with displacement of the anterior optic path-

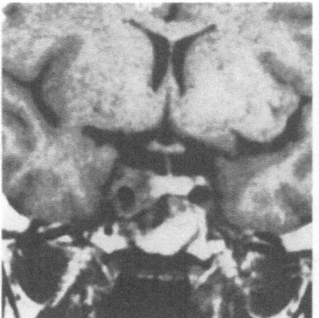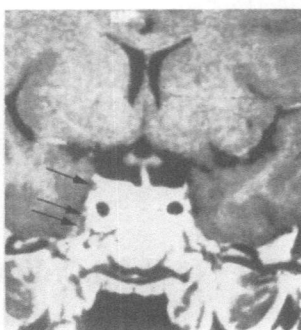

Fig. 1. Coronal MRI section of a recurrent pituitary adenoma on the right side: The recurrent tumour surrounds the "intracavernous" carotid artery, thus making surgical cure unlikely. The unenhanced scan (left) provides a better delineation of the almost normal pituitary gland from the tumour. This patient would be an ideal candidate for focused radiation therapy because: the optic pathways are far from the target, there is a clear margin to the normal pituitary gland, there is an exact delineation of the oculomotor nerve (arrow) as well as the trigeminal nerve (double arrow) within the lateral wall of the space of the cavernous sinus

ways . If the neurological situation allows, the management of choice is short term medical pretreatment to shrink the tumour followed by surgery to reduce the tumour bulk and then in most cases by adjuvant medical therapy [6, 14]. Frequently these tumours show diffuse invasion (= more than one area) which makes residual tumour more likely. In the case of drug intolerance, and in cases of tumour growth despite medication, radiation therapy may be indicated. Multilocular (parasellar, suprasellar, subsellar) invasion with or without residual tumour visible in MRI would allow focused radiation therapy less chance of a cure than with conventional radiation therapy. Unilocular residual tumour away from the visual pathways and the hypothalamus would be more suitable for focused radiation therapy. The question remains, whether the radiologically visible part alone is responsible for peristant homonal hypersecretion.

Growth Hormone Secreting Adenomas

As primary treatment, surgery can offer a chance of 70–90% cure in GH-microadenomas [2, 40]. In invasive and/or macroadenomas the surgical cure rate drops significantly [9]. Focused radiation therapy however seems to be relatively ineffective as only 2 of 7 previously untreated cases could be cured, and in 50% of all cases there was no, or only a minor effect [37]. Conventional radiation therapy takes 5 years to be effective with a 50–70% rate of pituitary insufficiency [7, 26, 34]. Medical treatment is available, but in regard to tumour shrinkage is not as effective as in the case of prolactinomas [18, 25].

Adrenocorticotropine Secreting Adenomas

Owing to the metabolic consequences, cure in Cushing's disease is mandatory and should be achieved without delay. Neurosurgery can offer a cure rate in 80–90% of patients [40]. Only in rare cases are diffuse invasive adenomas encountered and thus the surgical failures are mainly due to incorrect diagnosis and the inability to find the adenoma.

Neuro-imaging can only localize the tumour correctly in about 40% of cases. However, the neurosurgical cure rates are independent of neuro-imaging. In contrast to this, focused radiation therapy would need a clear (and correctly localized) target to be effective, although "blind" tratment had been reportedly performed [5, 30]. The success rate is reported to be 48% after a single dose and 76% after multiple irradiations with this treatment modality. With conventional radiation therapy however, the success of treatment will come too late for many patients. Although again in focused radiation therapy a long interval between treatment and relief from hypersecretion is also reported [5, 30].

Non-Secreting Adenomas

Due to late diagnosis, tumours are large and often invasive. Most cases have a chiasmal syndrome at diagnosis. Medical treatment is ineffective in most cases [25]. Surgery is the treatment of choice. Due to size and invasiveness residual tumour is frequently found. Only by repeated imaging studies–preferably with MRI–can tumour regrowth be proven. A determination of growth rate–as demonstrated by mAb KI-67 can give an idea of the velocity of expected regrowth [16, 20]. Depending on the growth rates of the residual tumour adjunctive therapy is needed. Not only the size and location of the residual tumour seems to be important in deciding, which form of radiation therapy should be given; since in many cases of macroadenomas the optic chiasma lowers down to the level of the diaphragma sellae or even below that level [36], and this may pose additional problems in the use of focused radiation therapy. Another fact of importance seems to be the occurrence of high proliferation rates

that have been found throughout the whole tumour and not just limited to the area, where the surgically or radiologically diagnosed invasion took place [15]. This fact implies that invasion is not a focal occurrence and it would also imply that a focal radiation treatment will not adequately deal with the problem.

Conclusion

There is undoubtably a need for adjunctive therapy in pituitary adenomas, especially in large, diffusely invasive adenomas which show high proliferation rates. In prolactinomas–regardless of the size–there is little or no need for focused radiation therapy; mainly because of the good results from medical treatment. Surgically treated acromegalic patients with parasellar residual tumour, would be the ideal candidates for focused radiation therapy, although the success rate is reported to be surprisingly low. In Cushing's disease current radiological techniques are only able to define the correct target for focused radiation therapy in less than 50% of cases and thus limiting the efficacy of this method.

References

1. Aubourg PR, Derome PJ, Peillon F, Jedynak CP, Visot A, Le Gentil P, Balagura S, Guiot G (1980) Endocrine outcome after transsphenoidal adenomectomy for prolactinoma: prolactin levels and tumour size as predicting factors. Surg Neurol 14: 141–143
2. Balagara S, Derome P, Guiot G (1981) Acromegaly: analysis of 132 cases treated surgically. Neurosurgery 8: 413–416
3. Barkan AL, Lloyd RV, Chandler WF (1988) Preoperative treatment of acromegaly with long-acting somatostatin analoge 201–995: shrinkage of invasive pituitary macroadenomas and improve surgical remission rate. J Clin Endocrin Metab 67: 1040–1048
4. Barrow DL, Mizuno J, Tindall GT (1988) Management of prolactinomas associated with very high serum prolactin levels. J Neurosurg 68: 554–558
5. Degerblad M, Rahn T, Bergstrand G, Thoren M (1986) Long-term results of stereotactic radiosurgery to the pituitary gland in Cushing's disease. Acta Endocrinol (Copenhagen) 112: 310–314
6. Fahlbusch R, Buchfelder M, Schrell U (1987) Short term pretreatment of macroprolactinomas by dopamin agonist. J Neurosurg 67: 807–815
7. Feek CM, McLelland J, Seth J, Toft AD, Irvine WJ, Padfield PL, Edwards CR (1984) How effective is external pituitary irradiation for growth hormone-secreting pituitary tumours? Clin Endocrinol (Oxford) 20: 401–408
8. Goodman ML (1990) Gamma knife radiosurgery: current status and review. South Med J 83: 551–554
9. Grisoli F, Leclercq T, Jaquet P, Guibout M, Winteler JP, Hassoun J, Vincentelli F (1985) Transsphenoidal surgery for acromegaly–long-term results in 100 patients. Surg Neurol 23: 513–519

10. Halberg FE, Sheline GE (1987) Radiotherapy of pituitary tumours. Endocrinol Metab Clin North Am 16: 667–684

11. Hardy J (1969) Transsphenoidal microsurgery of the normal and pathological pituitary. Clin Neurosurg 16: 185–217

12. Hardy J, Vezina JL (1976) Transsphenoidal neurosurgery of intracranial neoplasm. In: Thompson RA, Green JR (eds) Advances in neurology, Ud15. Raven, New York 15: 261–275

13. Hardy J (1983) Transsphenoidal microsurgery of prolactinomas: report on 355 cases. In: Tollis G, Stefanis C, Mountokalakis T (eds) Prolactin and prolactinomas. Raven, New York, pp 431–440

14. Hubbard JL, Scheithauer B, Abbound CF, Laws ER (1987) Prolactin secreting adenomas: the preoperative response to bromocryptine treatment and surgical outcome. J Neurosurg 67: 816–821

15. Kitz K, Knosp E, Korn A, Koos WTH (1991) Proliferation rate in 120 pituitary adenomas: measurement by mAb Ki-67. Acta Neurochir (Wien) [Suppl] 53: 60–64

16. Knosp E, Kitz K, Perneczky A (1989) Proliferation activity in pituitary adenomas: Measurement by monoclonal antibody Ki-67. Neurosurgery 25: 927–930

17. Knosp E, Steiner E, Kitz K (1993) Pituitary adenomas with invasion into the space of the cavernous sinus: an MRI classification compared with surgical findings. Neurosurgery 33: 610–618

18. Lamberts SWJ, Kitterlinden P, Schnieff PC, Klijnj GM (1988) Therapy of acromegaly with Sandostatin. Clin Endocrinol (Oxford) 29: 411–420

19. Landolt AM (1980) Biology of pituitary microadenomas. In: Faglia G, Giovanelli MA, Mac Leod RM (eds) Pituitary microadenomas. Academic Press, London pp 107–122

20. Landolt AM, Shibata T, Kleihues P (1987) Growth rate of human pituitary adenomas. J Neurosurg 67: 803–806

21. Landolt AM, Shibata T (1991) Growth, Cell Proliferation, and Prognosis of Pituitary Adenomas. In: Faglia G, Beck-Peccoz P, Ambrosi B, Travaglini P, Spada A (eds) Pituitary adenomas. New trends in basic and clinical research. Elsevier, New York, pp 169–178

22. Laws ER (1984) The neurosurgical management of acromegaly. In: Secretory tumours of the pituitary gland. In: Black McL, Zervas NT, Ridgeway EC, Martin JB (eds) Raven, New York, pp 169–173

23. Laws ER, Piepgras DG, Rendall RV (1979) Neurosurgical management of acromegaly. Results in 82 patients treated between 1972–1977. J Neurosurg 50: 454–461

24. Laws ER (1982) Transsphenoidal approach to lesions in and about the sella turcia. In: Schmidek KH, Sweet WH (eds) Current techniques in operative neurosurgery. Grune and Stratton, New York

25. Liuzzi A, Dallabonzana D, Oppizzi G, Arrigoni GL, Cozzi R, Strada S, Benini Z, Chiodini J, Chiodini PG (1991) Is there a real medical treatment for "non secreting" pituitary adenomas? In: Faglia G, Beck-Peccoz P, Ambrosi A, Travaglini P, Spada A (eds) Pituitary adenomas. New trends in basic and clinical research. Elsevier, New York pp 383–390

26. Lüdecke DK, Lutz BS, Niedworok G (1989) The choice of treatment after incomplete adenomectomy in acromegaly: proton-versus high voltage radiation. Acta Neurochir (Wien) 96: 32–38

27. Lunsford LD, Flickinger J, Coffey FJ (1990) Stereotactic gamma knife radiosurgery. Initial North American experience in 207 patients. Arch Neurol 47: 169–175

28. Martins AN, Hayes GJ, Kempe LG (1965) Invasive pituitary adenomas. J Neurosurg 22: 268–276

29. Quabbe HJ, Plöckinger U (1989) Dose-response study and long-term effect on the somatostatin analoge octreotide in patients with therapy-resistant acromegaly. J Clin Endocr Metab 68: 873–881

30. Rähn T, Thoren M, Hall K, Backlund EO (1980) Stereotactic radiosurgery in Cushing's syndrome: actute radiation effects. Surg Neurol 14: 85–92

31. Ross DA, Wilson CB (1988) Results of transsphenodial microsurgery for growth hormone-secreting pituitary adenomas in a series of 214 patients. J Neurosurg 68: 854–867

32. Scheithauer BS, Kovacs KT, Laws ER, Randall RV (1986) Pathology of invasive pituitary tumors with special reference to functional classification. J Neurosurg 65: 733–744

33. Selman WR, Laws ER, Scheithauer BW, Carpenter SM (1986) The occurrence of dural invasion in pituitary adenomas. J Neurosurg 64: 402–408

34. Snyder PJ, Fowble BF, Schatz JN, Savino PJ, Gennarelli TA (1986) Hypopituitarism following radiation therapy of pituitary adenomas. Am J Med 81: 457–462

35. Svoboda T, Luger A. Knosp E, Geyer G (1991) Prolactinom-Behandlung mit einem neuen Dopaminagonisten. Dtsch Med Wschr 116: 1224–1227

36. Steiner E, Knosp E, Herold CH, Kramer J, Stiglbauer R, Staniszewieski K, Imhof HJ (1992) Pituitary adenomas: findings of postoperative MR imaging. Radiology 185: 521–527

37. Thoren M, Rahn T, Hallengren B, Kaad PH, Nilsson KO, Ravn H, Ritzen M, Petersen KE, Aarskog D (1986) Treatment of Cushing's disease in childhood and adolescence by sterotactic pituitary irradiation. Acta Paediatr Scand 75: 388–395

38. Tindall GT, Tindall SC (1984) Transsphenoidal surgery for acromegaly: long term results in 50 patients In: Black McL, Zervas NT, Ridgemway EC, Martin JB (eds) Secretory tumors of the pituitary gland. Raven, New York, pp 175–178

39. Werder KV, Fahlbusch R, Landgraf R, Pichardt CR, Rjosk HK, Scriba PC (1978) Treatment of patients with prolactinomas. J Endocrinol Invest 1: 47–58

40. Wilson CHB (1984) A decade of pituitary microsurgery. The Herbert Olivecrona lecture. J Neurosurg 61: 814–834

41. Wrightson PH (1978) Conservative removal of small pituitary tumors: is it justified by the pathological findings? J Neurol Neurosurg Psychiatry 41: 283–289

Correspondence: E. Knosp, M. D., Neurochirurgische Abteilung, Sozialmedizinisches Zentrum Ost, Langobardenstr. 122, A-1220 Wien, Austria.

Acta Neurochir (1995) [Suppl] 63: 85–88

Gamma Knife Radiosurgery for Metastatic Brain Tumors

R. W. Rand, D. B. Jacques, R. W. Melbye, B. G. Copcutt, and **L. Irwin**

Johne Wayne Cancer Institute, Saint John's Hospital, Santa Monica, CA, U.S.A.

Summary

Sixty-three patients with metastatic brain tumors have had stereotactic radiosurgery 90 times with the Leksell Gamma Knife over a 29-month period. Initially, a single treatment of 35 to 45 Gy was delivered to the enhanced CT margin. This dose was found to be inadequate for tumor control. We then raised the marginal dose to 50 to 55 Gy, but even this radiosurgical dose did not appear to control tumor growth. However, we have found that metastatic brain tumors can be controlled successfully using enhanced MR scans and a peripheral dose of 60 Gy or even 65 Gy adjacent to the enhanced margins of the metastatic brain tumors, especially melanomas.

Keywords: Gamma knife; stereotactic radiosurgery; metastatic brain tumors.

Introduction

Brain metastases from malignancies of the lung, breast, skin melanoma, and kidney occur frequently in medical-surgical oncology patients. At least twenty percent or more of these cancer patients will be confronted with potentially lethal brain metastases [3, 7, 8, 10]. Conventional whole brain radiation alone has had disappointing results unless the metastatic cancers are quite small [6]. Therefore, stereotactic radiosurgery has been introduced to deliver a more intense and precise lethal treatment to these metastases [1, 2, 4, 5].

The concept of stereotactic radiosurgery was introduced by Professor Lars Leksell in 1951. A physicist colleague Professor Börje Larsson participated in the final version of the Gamma Knife, which is now celebrating 25 years of clinical use.

Materials and Methods

The Leksell Gamma Knife is ideal for treating brain metastases. The current Leksell Unit focuses 201 cobalt gamma beams to a central point within the shielded chamber. The size and shape of the radiation spheres are controlled by collimators of 4, 8, 14, and 18 mm. sized holes. The metastatic cancers can be detected with high-resolution contrast CT and MRI imaging even when they are relatively small. In addition, the tumor margins of metastases are easier to identify than the tumor margins of primary gliomas because the metastases do not tend to invade the brain tissues as much as primary gliomas.

From March 1991 through August 1993, the Leksell Gamma Knife at the Hospital of the Good Samaritan in Los Angeles was used 90 times to treat 63 patients with brain metastases (Table 1). Several of these patients have had more than one Gamma Knife treatment, either because all of the metastases could not be fitted within the original stereotactic space of the Leksell frame, or because the metastases showed evidence of further growth.

Originally, CT scans with intravenous iodine enhancement were employed. However, we changed to using MRI scans once we were able to develop precise MRI coordinates with the introduction of special head fixation and head coils, which eliminated magnetic field distortion of the coordinates. Now, we use enhanced MRI scans exclusively, unless there are some specific contraindications such as a cardiac pacemaker, metal aneurysm clips, etc.

We have changed the treatment plans over the past two years, as shown in the following case studies.

Patient 1

An early patient had a single metastatic tumor of renal origin in the cerebellum. The metastatic tumor had been previously treated by 4,000 rads of whole brain radiation, but tumor growth was not controlled. He underwent stereotactic radiosurgery, and 35 Gy were delivered to the tumor margin imaged by enhanced CT. A second stereotactic radiosurgical operation was performed four months later using 45 Gy at the tumor margin because of continued growth of the metastasis. Despite these two radiosurgical operations, the tumor grew uncontrollably. The patient died ten months later because of widespread cancer in the abdomen and increased intracranial pressure from the cerebellar metastasis.

Patient 2

An elderly lung cancer patient had two metastatic neoplasms, one in the right parietal lobe and the other in the left centrum near the

Table 1. *Patients with Metastatic Brain Tumors Treated with the Gamma Knife from March 1991 Through August 1993 at the Hospital of the Good Samaritan in Los Angeles*

Source of metastasis	Number of patients	Number of Gamma Knife treatments
Breast	4	6
Colon	1	1
Endometrial	1	1
Lung	25	32
Melanoma	23	36
Ovarian	1	2
Renal	3	5
Squamous cell	1	1
Thyroid	1	1
Unknown	3	5
Total	63	90

midline. The patient underwent Gamma Knife radiosurgical treatment, which was well tolerated under local anesthetic. The right parietal tumor received 55 Gy at the margin, as identified by enhanced CT. The parasaggital metastatic tumor received 60 Gy at the margin. Follow-up films demonstrated that the parietal tumor, which received 55 Gy, continued to grow and the growth of the other tumor, which received 60 Gy, was arrested. The patient died of pneumonia during radiation of her lung cancer. The patient's family did not consent to an autopsy.

Patient 3

Another example is a 50-year-old woman with four metastatic neoplasms, one in the left occipital lobe, a second in the right occipital lobe, a third in the left frontal lobe, and a fourth adjacent to the lateral ventricle, all of which were probably from primary lung cancer. Each tumor was treated with 60 Gy near the margin of the tumor as shown by Gadolinium-enhanced MRI.

Following stereotactic radiosurgery, a stereotactic biopsy of the left occipital tumor was obtained uneventfully. The biopsy demonstrated that the neoplasm was an adenocarcinoma. Because of the apparent continued growth of two of the metastases, the patient received additional radiosurgery using a radiation dose of 65 Gy to the margin of the enhanced MR tumor scans. These two tumors have shown no further growth, and radionecrosis has occurred. In retrospect, the original treatment dose of 60 Gy was sufficient to destroy these tumors. Meanwhile, the other smaller metastases have disappeared.

Patient 4

The last example is a 52-year-old woman with prior mastectomy for breast cancer. It was discovered that she had a metastatic tumor in the cerebellum. The patient had no prior radiation therapy to the brain, and a stereotactic radiosurgical procedure was planned. The enhanced MR images with the Leksell frame in place revealed three additional metastatic brain tumors. Each of the four tumors was treated by a single Gamma Knife radiosurgical dose of 60 Gy to the enhanced tumor margin. Follow-up MR films three months later showed no further growth of these tumors. In fact, the cerebellar tumor had decreased significantly in size.

Results

It became apparent from our clinical cases that the originally recommended peripheral focused radiosurgical dose of 35 to 45 Gy to the margin of the metastatic tumors appeared to be inadequate to control growth and recurrence. We have found that a marginal dose of 50 to 55 Gy also appeared to be inadequate to destroy these cancers. Therefore, we have concluded that, whenever possible, the single radiosurgical treatment dose plan should be in the range of 60 Gy or even 65 Gy at the enhanced margin of the tumor. CT enhanced images do not represent the true tumor margin. Therefore, we now use triple enhanced MR images in every patient unless there is a specific contraindication because the tumor margin can be more exactly demonstrated. Figures 1a and b, 2a and b, 3a and b represent current results using this stereotactic radiation dose planning.

We have been able to follow 56 metastatic melanoma brain tumors with MRI scans for one to six months after treatment. Sixteen tumors have disappeared completely; 26 neoplasms were smaller; and fourteen tumors were the same size. Thus, Gamma Knife radiosurgery has resulted in a virtually 100% melanoma control rate.

Except for two melanomas near the brain stem, all of the metastatic melanomas were treated with 60–65 Gy to the 50% isodose line at least to the enhanced tumor margins. One quite small tumor near the brain stem received 40 Gy, and the other larger metastasis near the brain stem received 20 Gy. The tumor that received

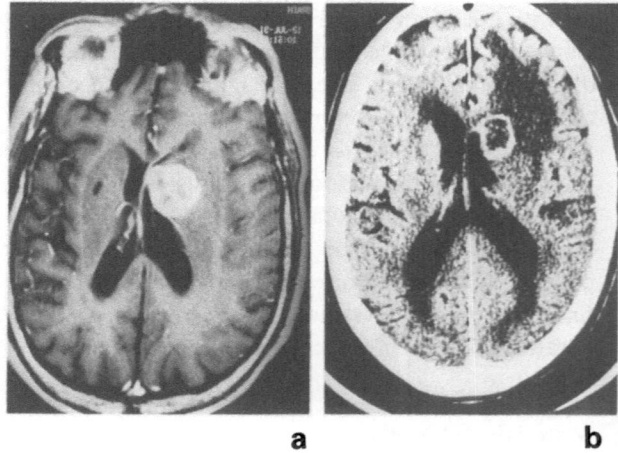

a   **b**

Fig. 1. (a) Large, single metastatic renal carcinoma. (b) Necrosis of the tumor following Gamma Knife stereotactic radiosurgery of 65 Gy at the margin

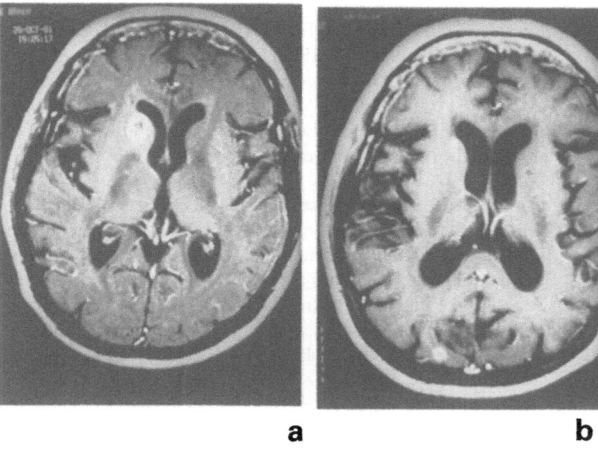

Fig. 2. (a) Solitary metastatic breast cancer tumor. (b) Necrosis of the cancer with 65 Gy at the margin using the Leksell Gamma Knife

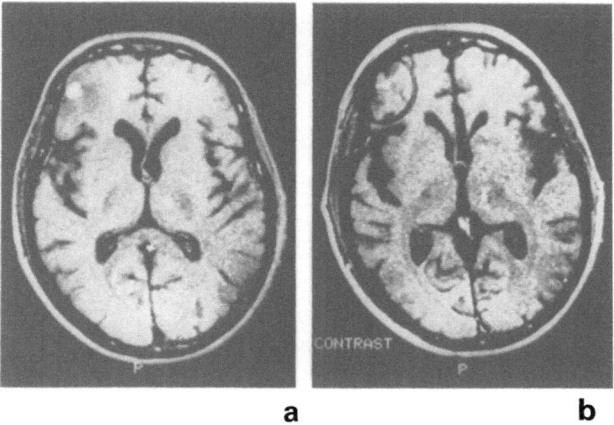

Fig. 3. (a) Metastatic melanoma in the right frontal lobe. (b) Necrosis achieved with 65 Gy at the margin using stereotactic radiosurgery with the Gamma Knife

only 20 Gy continued to grow and required surgical resection. Viable tumor cells undergoing mitosis were found in the peripheral areas of the tumor.

Discussion

The survival period of patients with untreated brain metastases is short, usually six months or less. Patients with a single metastasis treated with open brain surgery and fractionated radiotherapy have longer useful survival periods than those treated with radiotherapy alone. However, many patients do not have surgically accessible metastases [7, 8]. Stereotactic radiosurgery

using the Leksell Gamma Knife offers these patients their best chance of prolonged survival if the treatment dose is lethal to the cancer cells [1, 2, 4, 9]. A high tumor response rate can be achieved by stereotactic radiosurgery with the Gamma Knife. Therefore, the quality of life as measured by Karnofsky score, neurologic function, and steroid dependence is improved.

In our opinion, it is necessary to employ higher doses of focused radiation than have generally been recommended and used by other radiosurgical facilities. Originally, we were advised that a single dose of 35 to 45 Gy was sufficient to control marginal metastatic tumor growth. However, all of our early patients who were treated with 35 to 45 Gy at the margin required retreatment to try to control continued metastatic tumor growth.

Therefore, after careful evaluation of our patients, we have come to the following specific conclusions: The margin dose of the metastatic neoplasms should be 60 Gy or even 65 Gy whenever possible, depending upon the location of vital structures, in order to destroy the single and multiple metastases with one treatment; CT scans, even with double contrast, may not accurately outline the size, shape, volume, or margins of metastatic tumors; and MR with triple constrast is a better method of scanning to determine size, shape, volume, and margins of these neoplasms. If CT enhanced images are used, the margin of therapy should be a few millimeters beyond the enhanced margin.

Special head coils and fixation are required to eliminate the magnetic-field distortions of MR scans in order to determine accurately the stereotactic x, y, and z coordinates. Newer types of Gadolinium compounds are superior in identifying cerebral metastases by MR enhanced images. An MRI with triple contrast should be performed one month after the Gamma Knife treatment to assess the benefit and to identify any new metastases that may need to be treated.

Patients with metastatic brain tumors are candidates for Gamma Knife stereotactic radiosurgery only if, in the opinion of their medical and surgical oncologists, they have reasonable survival opportunities. Patients treated with Gamma Knife stereotactic radiosurgery should continue with appropriate medical and surgical therapy to control systemic disease.

Acknowledgment

The authors are grateful to Betty Day for providing all of the photographs.

References

1. Adler JR, Cox RS, Kaplan I (1992) Stereotactic radiosurgical treatment of brain metastases. J Neurosurg 76: 444–449
2. Alexander E III, Loeffler JS (1992) Radiosurgery using a modified linear accelerator. Neurosurg Clin North Am 3: 167–190
3. Buckner J (1992) Surgery, radiation therapy, and chemotherapy for metastatic tumors to the brain. Curr Opin Oncol 4: 518–524
4. Caron JL, Souhami L, Podgorsak EB (1992) Dynamic stereotactic radiosurgery in the palliative treatment of cerebral metastatic tumors. J Neurooncol 12: 173–179
5. Coffey RJ, Lunsford LD, Flickinger JC (1992) The role of radiosurgery in the treatment of malignant brain tumors. Neurosurg Clin North Am 3: 231–244
6. Fuller BG, Kaplan ID, Adler J (1992) Stereotaxic radiosurgery for brain metastases: the importance of adjuvant whole brain irradiation. Int J Radiation Oncol Biol Phys 23: 413–418
7. Mehta MP, Rosenthal JM, Levin AB, Mackie TR, Kubsad SS, Gehring MA, Kinsella TJ (1992) Defining the role of radiosurgery in the management of brain metastases. Int J Radiation Oncol Biol Phys 24: 619–625
8. Patchell RA, Tibbs PA, Walsh JW (1990) A randomized trial of surgery in the treatment of single metastases to the brain. N Engl J Med 322: 494–500
9. Strum V, Kimmig B, Engenhardt R, Schlegel W, Pastyr O, Treuer H, Schabbert S, Voges J (1991) Radiosurgical treatment of cerebral metastases: method, indications and results. Stereotact Funct Neurosurg 57: 7–10
10. Tsukada Y, Fouad A, Pickren JW, Lane WW (1983) Central nervous system metastasis from breast carcinoma: autopsy study. Cancer 52: 2349–2354

Correspondence: Robert W. Rand, Ph.D., M.D. John Wayne Cancer Institute, Saint John's Hospital and Health Center 1328 Twenty-Second Street Santa Monica, CA 90404, U.S.A.

Acta Neurochir (1995) [Suppl] 63: 89–94

Radiosurgery of the Metastatic Brain Tumours with Gamma-Knife

Y. Kida, T. Kobayashi, and **T. Tanaka**

Department of Neurosurgery, Komaki City Hospital, Jhobusi, Komaki, Japan

Summary

The results of treatment of metastatic brain tumours by radiosurgery are reported. Twenty cases including lung (11), colon (5), breast (1), ovary (1), liver cancer (1) and malignant melanoma (1) were involved. Seven cases had single and 13 had multiple brain metastases. In total 55 lesions were evaluated after radiosurgery with the gamma-knife. Following localization with MR1 and dose planning, radiosurgery with marginal doses between 12 to 25 Gy (mean 18.9 Gy) was delivered. In the follow-up studies with MRI after 3 months, 29 out of 55 (52.7%) lesions showed significant shrinkage. In contrast 25 showed either no change (17) or central necrosis (8), and one was enlarged. Thus the tumour control at 3 months was 98.2%, and subsequently 96.6% at 6 months. Clinical symptoms and signs were improved in most cases, but were aggravated in four cases either by tumour recurrence or by radiation-induced oedema. Although the tumours treated with radiosurgery were well controlled, tumour recurrence in another sites occurred in 4 case, of which 3 were treated by 2nd radiosurgery with 2 successful tumour control. Complications were generally mild and transient. In summary stereotactic radiosurgery is valuable new treatment not only for solitary metastases, but also for multiple or recurrent ones.

Keywords: Metastatic brain tumours; radiosurgery; gamma knife.

Introduction

In the treatment of metastatic brain tumour, one of the most important tasks for the neurosurgeon is to completely control the tumour growth and to guarantee a good quality of life for those patients. Since brain metastases are generally well-circumscribed and relatively small in size, stereotactic radiosurgery seems to be one of the possible alternatives to currently used treatment modalities i.e. operation, chemotherapy or conventional radiotherapy. With stereotactic radiosurgery focused irradiation to the target volume can be done by its steep dose gradients without damaging surrounding brain tissue [5, 6]. There have been only a few reports on the radiosurgery of brain metastases in

the past [1, 7, 9, 11, 12]. We have installed the gamma-knife on May 1991 and already treated more than 400 cases including cerebral AVM, acoustic tumours, meningiomas as well as metastatic brain tumours. In this paper the responses of metastatic brain tumors to radiosurgery are reported in order to see whether they are suitable for this treatment and how they can be controlled.

Materials and Methods

The gamma-knife, containing 201 Co-60 sources can deliver focused irradiation with sharp falling-off through the collimator. Currently four different sizes of collimator, 4, 8, 14 and 18 mm in diameter were used alone or in combination, depending on the target volume and the shape. After firmly fixing the Leksell's Stereotactic Frame to the head, imaging studies with CT or MRI were performed for the localization of lesions. Then the computerized dosimetry was carried out, followed by stereotactic radiosurgery using the gamma-knife. Except for a few cases the enhanced T1-weighted image of MRI was used for localization as shown in Fig. 1. Both axial and coronal images were used for the dosimetry so as to be matched with the spacial configuration of the tumour.

From May 1991 to August 1992, 20 cases of metastatic brain tumour were treated by gamma-knife, of whom 11 cases came from lung cancer, 5 from colon, one each from breast, ovary and the liver, and one malignant melanoma was included. Histologically all but one (malignant melanoma) were adenocarcinomas. Seven cases had single and 13 had multiple metastases when treated. In total 55 metastatic tumours (mean 2.7 tumours per case) were involved. There were 12 males and 8 females, whose ages ranged from 27 to 77., with an average of 59.2. Eight out of 20 cases had external irradiation before radiosurgery, and another 2 cases received it after radiosurgery. The other 10 cases were treated by radiosurgery alone and had no external irradiation (Table 1).

Follow-up studies were made every three months with evaluation of the neurological condition and of CT or MRI. The mean diameter of the tumours were compared with the ones prior to radiosurgery and were classified in terms of CR (Complete Remission – disappearance of the tumour), PR (partial remission – tumour shrinkage more than 50%), MR (minor response – tumour shrinkage between 25 to

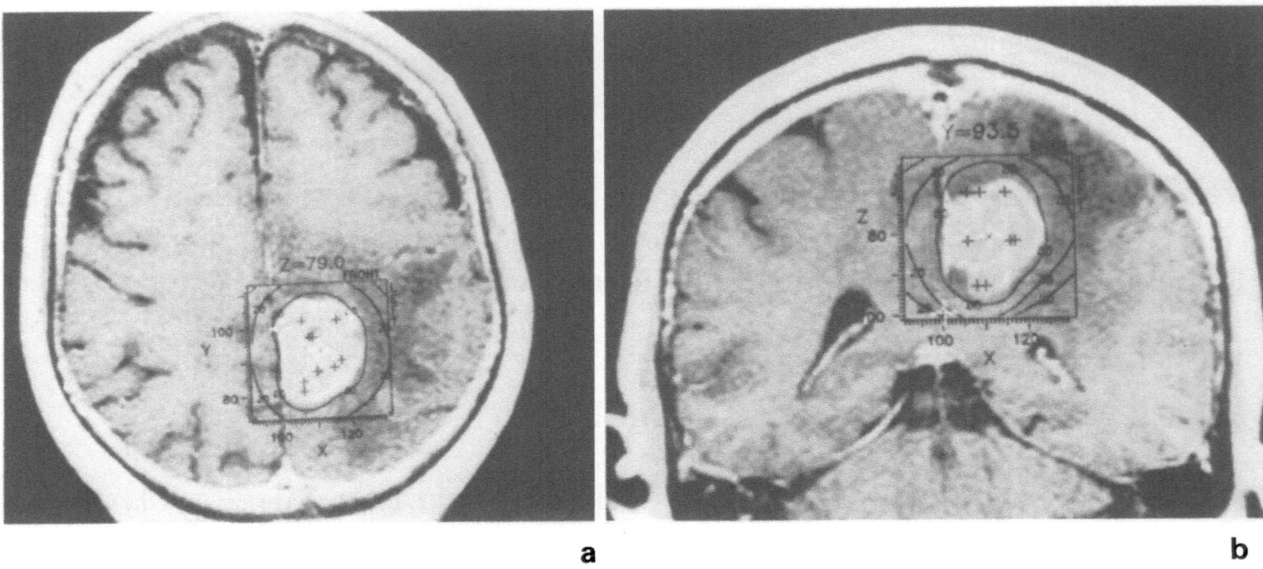

Fig. 1. Localization of brain metastasis with T1-enhanced MRI is shown. (a) Axial. (b) Coronal

Table 1. *Patient Characteristics*

No. of patients	20
Male	12
Female	8
Age distribution	27 to 77 years
Average	59.2 years
Primary site, histology, lesions ( )	
Lung adenocarcinoma	11 (29)
Colon adenocarcinoma	5 (13)
Breast adenocarcinoma	1 (1)
Ovary adenocarcinoma	1 (3)
Liver adenocarcinoma	1 (1)
Malignant melanoma	1 (8)
Multiplicity	
Single metastasis	7
Multiple metastases	13

50%), NC (no change – change of tumour diameter between 25 to −25%) and PG (progression-tumour enlarged more than 25%). Length of survival and the rate of brain tumour control after radiosurgery were also investigated.

Results

The summary of the treatment dose in relation to the tumour size are demonstrated in the Table 2. The majority of the tumours were less than 20 mm in mean diameter and only one lesion was larger than 30 mm. In radiosurgery, tumours were treated with 17 to 44 Gy of maximum doses, and with 14 to 25.2 Gy of marginal doses. Most of the tumours were treated by nearly 20 Gy at the margins, with an average of 18.9 Gy. However it was reduced sometimes below 16 Gy depending on the tumour size and its location. Currently marginal doses were set exclusively on the 50% isodose line or more of the maximum (100%) doses, but in three tumours it was less than 50%. 3 months after radiosurgery, 11 tumours disappeared (CR), 18 significantly reduced (PR + MR) and 25 showed no change in size, in which 8 tumours demonstrated apparent low signal intensity centrally, indicating central necrosis. Only

Table 2

Radiosurgery of metastatic brain tumours (55 lesions)				Marginal doses for brain metastases			
Size of tumour	Lesions	Max. dose	Marg. dose (mean)	(20 cases − 55 lesions)			
1 0–10 mm	19	17–40 Gy	15–25.2 (19.2) Gy	40%	1	60%	4
2 10–15	8	30–41	18–25.0 (21.8)	45%	2	70%	4
3 15–20	13	30–40	15–25.0 (19.2)	50%	41	80%	0
4 20–25	6	30–40	15–20.0 (17.2)	55%	1	90%	2
5 25–30	8	28–44	14–20.0 (17.0)				
6 30–35	1	24	12 (12.0)				
Mean	55	17–44	12–25.2 (18.9)				

one tumour enlarged after the treatment. Thus 29 out of 55 (52.7%) showed a good response, and 54 out of 55 tumours (98.2%) were well controlled at the 3rd month. Similarly more than 80% of the tumours those which were seen at 6 and 9 months follow-up, were controlled (Table 3). It is noted that such remarkable responses could often be seen in the early few months after radiosurgery (Fig. 2). The relationship between tumour size, marginal dose and the response at 3 months is illustrated in Fig. 3. More than half of the metastases significantly reduced in size or disappeared. It is apparent that smaller tumours tend to disappear faster than larger ones.

Prognosis of the 20 patients is shown in Table 4. Neurologically many of the patients showed consider-

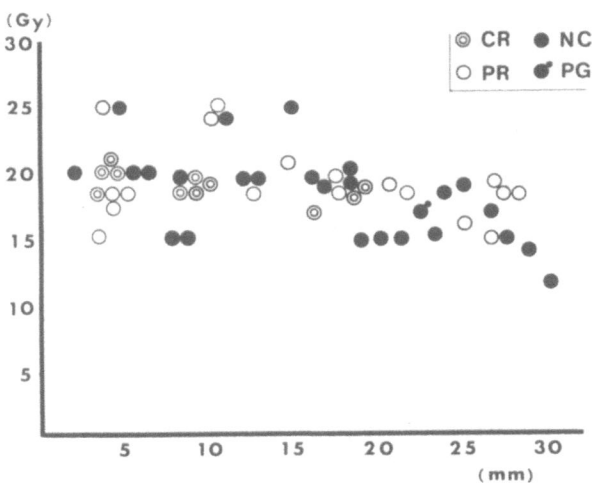

Fig. 3. Scattergram of marginal dose versus mean diameter of brain metastases. The responses of tumours at 3 month are demonstrated as CR (Complete Remission) (◎), PR (Partial Remission) + MR (Minor Response) (○), NC (No Change) (●) and PG (Progression) (●*). More than half of the tumours show significant tumour shrinkage.

Table 3. *Follow-up Results on MRI or CT (55 Lesions)*

	3M	6M	9M
Disappeared	11	7	3
Decreased in size	18	9	3
Central necrosis	8	4	2
No change	17	8	0
Enlarged	1	1	2
Total	55	29	10

Table 4. *Outcome of Patients (20 Cases of Brain Metastases)*

A. Clinical symptoms and signs	
Complete regression	2
Partial regression	10
No change	4
Worsened	4
Tumour progression	2
Radiation-induced oedema	2
B. Prognosis	
Dead 10 (mean survival after RS: 6.4 M)	
Cause of death	
Brain metastasis	1
Spinal cord meta	2
Primary cancer	5
Cerebral haemorrhage	1
Heart attack	1
Alive 10 (mean follow-up after RS: 8.3 M)	
Brain tumour control	
Excellent	8
Poor	1
Unknown	1
Recurrence at another site	4

RS radiosurgery.

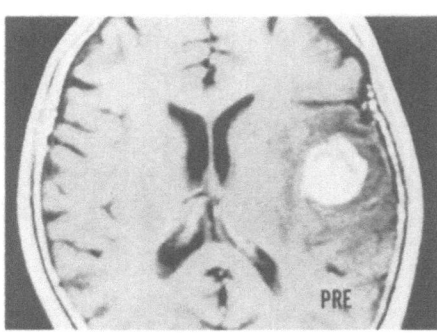
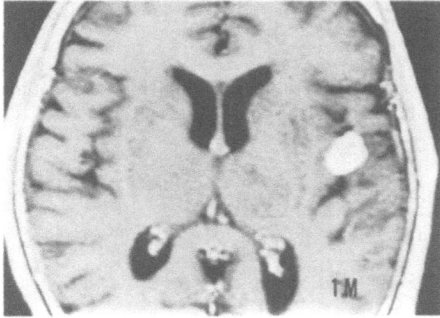

Fig. 2. Early responses of metastatic tumour from cancer of the colon are demonstrated (1 month after the radiosurgery). Not only the tumour regression, but also marked decrease of perifocal oedema is noted

able improvement. Complete regression of symptoms was obtained in 2, partial regression in 10 and no remarkable changes in 4 cases. However, 4 cases showed deterioration of their neurological condition due to tumour progression in 2, radiation-induced perifocal oedema in 2. Currently 10 patients had already died and the mean survival period after radiosurgery was 6.4 months. The cause of death was brain metastasis in 1 case, spinal cord metastases in two, cerebral haemorrhage from tumour in 1 and heart attack in one. Another 5 cases died because of progression of their primary cancer. Except for 2 cases, the tumours treated by radiosurgery were well controlled until death. The other 10 cases are still alive with 8.3 months of mean follow-up period. The control of brain metastases treated by radiosurgery was excellent in 8, poor in 1 and unknown in 1. Unfortunately tumour recurrence occurred in other sites of the brain in 4 cases.

Retreatment with Radiosurgery

Recurrence of brain metastases in other sites occurred in 4 cases, of whom 3 were treated by radiosurgery again with intervals of 2, 3 and 4 months respectively. Successful tumour control was achieved in 2 of them without any adverse effect (Table 5). Figure 4 shows an example of favourable response of brain metastases to initial as well as repeated radiosurgery.

Adverse Effects

No systemic or neurological complications occurred during or just after the radiosurgery. Radiation-in-duced oedema was observed in three cases, in whom two were symptomatic and required medication with corticosteroids for several weeks. The symptoms were generally mild and fully recovered.

Illustrative Cases

A 63 year old woman (breast cancer). This 63-year-old woman had been suffering from breast cancer since 1989, developed weakness of the left arm and leg. Because of continued deterioration, she was referred to us for radiosurgery. Her CT scan on admission disclosed a small tumour, 2 cm in diameter, involving the right cerebral peduncle. On July 23, 1991, she was treated by radiosurgery at a dose of 18 Gy at the tumour margin, which represents 60% isodose of the maximum dose. During the following 3 months, her neurological signs were well improved and her CT scan showed a marked shrinkage of the tumour (Fig. 5). Then her general condition became worse because of progression of lung metastases and she died of respiratory distress in October 1991. No tumour recurrence was seen in the brain at that time.

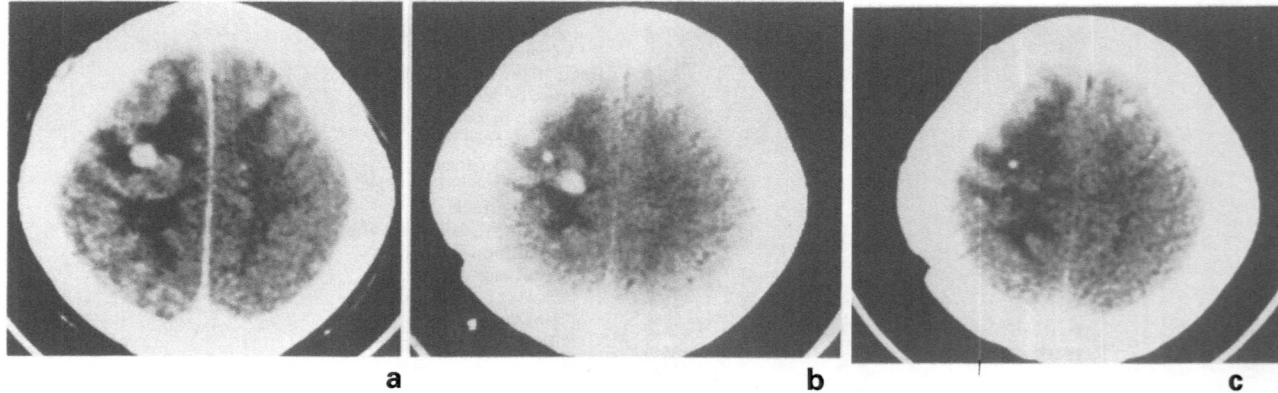

Fig. 4. Metastatic tumours from the colon were initially treated by radiosurgery (25 Gy at the margins) (a). The recurrent tumour (b) was treated again by radiosurgery (25 Gy at the margin) 3 months later and successful tumour control was obtained (c)

Table 5. *Retreatment of Brain Metastases by Radiosurgery*

	Case	1st Rs	Result	Interval	2nd Rs	Result
1	Colon	2 (25 Gy)	2 PR	3 M	1 (25 Gy)	1 CR
2	Lung	3 (17–21)	2 PR 1 PG	2 M	3 (18 Gy)	2 PR 1 NC
3	Colon	5 (17–20)	5 CR	4 M	4 (20 Gy)	NV

RS radiosurgery, *NV* not verified, *CR* complete remission, *PR* partial remission, *NC* no change, *PG* progression.

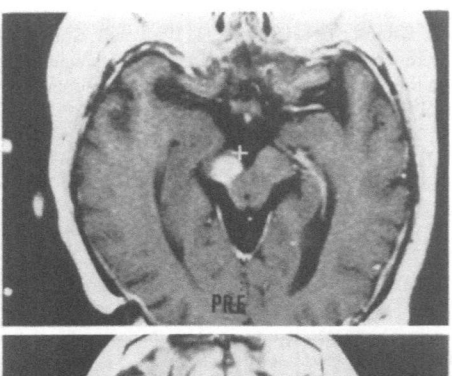

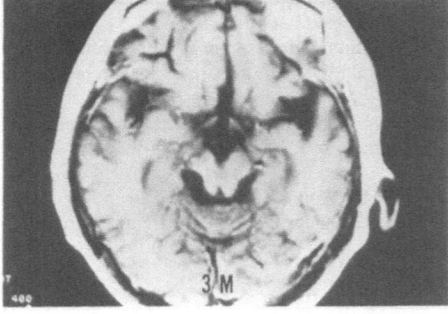

Fig. 5. Case 1. A solitary brain metastasis from a cancer of the breast in right cerebral peduncle shows a marked shrinkage 3 months after radiosurgery (18 Gy at the margin)

A 63 year old woman (ovarian cancer). This is the case with multiple brain metastases from ovarian papillary adenocarcinoma. All the 3 metastases in the brain stem and cerebellum were treated by radiosurgery with marginal doses of 15 to 20 Gy. The tumours showed a moderate response as early as 1 month and consistent regression subsequently (Fig. 6). Although

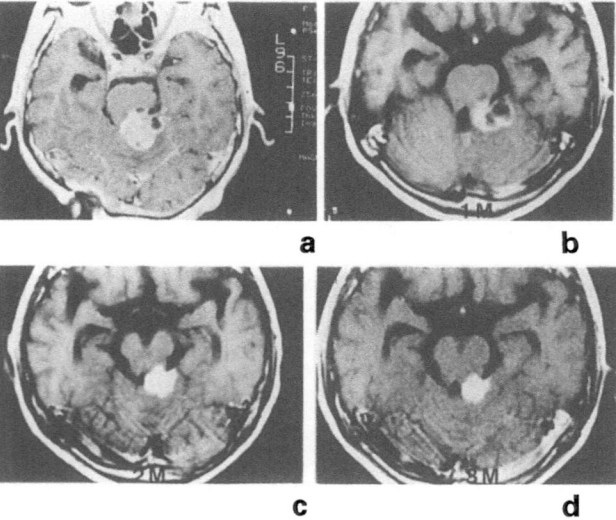

Fig. 6. Case 2. Multiple brain metastases from ovarian cancer to brain stem and cerebellum demonstrate considerable shrinkage after radiosurgery (15–20 Gy at the margins). Each MRI represents before (a) and 1 (b), 2 (c), 3 (d) months following treatment respectively

she recovered well from brain stem symptoms and signs, she died of spinal cord metastases 6 month later.

Discussion

There are various problems in the treatment of metastatic brain tumours. In general a single metastasis is currently treated by an operative procedure when they are resectable. If they are multiple or surgically unresectable, conventional radiotherapy or chemotherapy are commonly selected. Recently radiosurgical approaches have been developed [5] and tried in several institutes [6, 8, 10]. A few studies on radiosurgery of metastatic brain tumours have been reported [7, 9, 11, 12]. The results seemed to be excellent and encouraging, but (including real indications) it has not been established as a new treatment modality. As shown in our cases, it is apparent that most of the brain metastases respond well to radiosurgery using the gamma-knife. Moreover the effects become apparent much faster and are more consistent than those of benign brain tumours like neurinoma [3] and meningioma [2, 4]. In fact more than half of the brain metastases demonstrated significant reduction in the enhancing volume in the first 3 months after radiosurgery. The marginal dose near 20 Gy seems to be adequate to control the tumour growth as well as to prevent radiation-related complications. As other investigators [11] noted, the complications occurred in the cases of large tumours treated with relatively high marginal doses. It is of great importance in radiosurgery of brain metastases not to cause symptomatic complications since they may disturb the patient's condition and thereby the quality of life. In this sense the tumour size which can be handled by radiosurgery should be less than 30 mm in mean diameter.

Larger tumours have to be treated by other treatment modalities or treated by radiosurgery after sufficient volume reduction of the tumour has been achieved. Treatment failures may occur in some, partly due to inadequate localization, low irradiation dose or to low sensitivity of the tumour. Dissemination of the tumour is one of the important causes of failure since this is so often obscured in imaging studies. Gliosis following operative procedures may also obscure the tumour margin and sometimes disturb the localization. There is another question whether multiple metastases can be handled by radiosurgery or not. Currently only the single metastasis has been considered as a proper indication for radiosurgery [12]. How-

ever even several metastases could be treated successfully in our series. Since the gamma-knife has the great
advantage of being able to move easily from one target
to the other, multiple metastases can be treated by
radiosurgery. Although radiosurgery can control the
tumour, it is impossible to prevent the recurrence of
brain metastassis at other sites. Whole brain irradiation may be required in those cases as other investigators [9] suggested. But the retreatment with
radiosurgery might be a choice because this can be
completed within a few days of admission.

Conclusion

More than half of the brain metastases treated using
the gamma-knife significantly reduced in size or disappeared within the first 3 months. The majority of them
could be well controlled subsequently, though another
brain metastasis may occur at another site. Multiple
metastases with at least several tumours can be treated
using the gamma-knife at the same time, and it can be
repeated when the tumours recurout at other sites. The
marginal doses between 15 to 25 Gy are apparently
effective for those tumours which are less than 30 mm
in mean diameter, and are usually safe for the surrounding brain.

References

1. Davey P, O Brien P (1991) Disposition of cerebral metastases
   from malignant melanoma: Implication for radiosurgery. Neurosurgery 28: 8–15

2. Engenhardt R, Kimmig BN, Hover KH, Wowra B, Sturm V,
   Kaick GV, Wannenmacher M (1990) Stereotactic single high
   dose radiation therapy of benign intracranial meningiomas. Int
   J Radiat Oncol Biol Phys 19: 1021–1026
3. Flickinger JC, Lunsford LD, Coffey RJ, Linsky ME, Bissonette
   DJ, Maitz AH, Kondziolka D (1991) Radiosurgery of acoustic
   neurinomas. Cancer 67: 345–353
4. Kondziolka D, Lunsford LD, Coffey RJ, Flickinger JC (1991)
   Stereotactic radiosurgery of meningiomas. J Neurosurg 74: 552–
   559
5. Leksell L (1951) The stereotactic method and radiosurgery of the
   brain. Acta Chir Scand 102: 316–319
6. Leksell DG (1987) Stereotactic radiosurgery: present status and
   future trends. Neuro Res 9: 60–68
7. Lindquist C (1989) Gamma knife surgery for recurrent solitary
   metastasis of a cerebral hypernephroma: case report. Neurosurgery 25: 802–804
8. Loeffler JS, Alexander E (1990) The role of stereotactic radiosurgery in the management of intracranial tumours. Oncology 4:
   21–41
9. Loeffler JS, Kooy HM, Wen PY, Fine HA, Cheng CW, Man-
   narino EG, Tsai JS, Alexander E (1990) The treatment of recurrent brain metastasis with stereotactic radiosurgery. J Clin
   Oncol 8: 576–582
10. Lunsford LD, Flickinger J, Coffey RJ (1990) Stereotactic gamma
    knife radiosurgery. Initial North American experience in 207
    patients. Acta Neurol 47: 169–175
11. Sturm V, Kober B, Hover KH, Schlegel W, Boesecke R,
    Pastyr O, Hartmann GH, Schabbert S, Winkel K, Kunze S,
    Lorenz WJ (1987) Stereotactic percutaneous single dose irradi-
    ation of brain metastases with a linear accelerator. Int J Radiat
    Oncol Biol Phys 13: 279–282
12. Sturm V, Kimmig B, Engenhardt R, Schlegel W, Pastyr
    O, Treuer H, Schabbert S, Voges J (1991) Radiosurgical treat-
    ment of cerebral metastases. Stereotact Funct Neurosurg 57:
    7–10

Correspondence: Yoshihisa Kida, M. D., Department of Neurosurgery, Komaki City Hospital, 1-20, Jhobusi, Komaki City, Aichi
Pref., Japan.

Acta Neurochir (1995) [Suppl] 63: 95–100

The Results of Radiosurgical Management of 139 Single Cerebral Metastases

V. Valentino

Centro di Radiochirurgia, Clinica Flaminia, Rome, Italy

Summary

Between March 1984 and June 1993, linac radiosurgery was performed in 139 patients for single brain metastases, using the non-invasive (Greitz-Bergström) head fixation system. This atraumatic system was utilized for subsequent stereotactic CT/NMR staging to obtain strictly comparable neuro-imaging. Thus, tumour response was evaluated precisely and radiosurgery repeated (straight after the diagnostic sitting), as needed. No hospitalization or anaesthesia was necessary.

The 25 mm target was the maximum size to avoid the risk of radiation induced reactions. In metastases exceeding this limit single doses were directed at more than one target at the same session. Focusing upon single or multiple targets was facilitated by 3-D stereotactic NMR. The results after one single sitting were compared with those obtained after staged sittings in the same patients. Radiosurgery achieved disappearance or shrinkage of the metastasis with resolution of the oedema and mid-line shift in 86% of the 139 patients treated. In 47% of them, however, the success was the result of repeat radiosurgery and staged sittings. The non-invasive procedure is the keystone to optimize the radiosurgical results.

Keywords: Radiosurgery; brain metastases; stereotaxis.

Introduction

It is known that the unfortunate patients struck by brain metastases are doomed to a short survival of 3–6 months. According to statistics no more than 5% have survived for longer than 2 years.

Neurosurgery can tackle solitary metastases on condition that (1) they are not deep-seated and do not involve vital neural structures; (2) the patient still has an acceptable Karnofsky performance status (KPS); and (3) other organs are not yet seriously involved. As an alternative to neurosurgery, a desperate resort to fractionated irradiation or chemotherapy is all that remains. However, the inefficacy of both these treatments of brain metastases has been proved equal to their neurotoxicity.

Just as for other malignant intracranial tumours, attempts have been made to perfect techniques able to benefit patients who have only a limited life expectancy. In the light of this bitter truth, the ideal (if such a term could be used) would be to help them suffer as little as possible, and ever since 1984 we have used non-traumatic stereotactic radiosurgery for patients with single cerebral metastases.

The aim of this study is to analyse the results of this technique in a series of 139 patients.

Patient Population

From March 1984 to June 1993, 1560 patients with intracranial tumours and AVMs underwent stereotactic radiosurgery in Rome (Centro di Radiochirurgia, Clinica Flaminia), 139 of whom had single cerebral metastases (Table 1). Seventy-eight of these patients were male and 61 female. The mean age was 50 years (range 19–79). Lung cancer was the primary tumour in 61 patients and breast cancer in 32. Other brain metastases were from malignant melanoma (8 patients), gastro-intestinal cancer (11 patients), urinary-tract cancer (10 patients) and osteosarcoma (1 patient). The primary tumour remained unknown in 16 patients. The patients were unselected, and the KPS ranged from 40–90 (median 65). In 110 patients the metastasis was supra-tentorial and in 29 it was infra-tentorial, involving the brain stem in 4 patients. Post-operative radiosurgery was performed in 20 patients after incomplete surgical removal of the metastasis (12 patients), or local recurrence (5 patients). In 3 patients the radiosurgical treatment was prophylactic to the tumour bed after an apparently complete removal of the metastasis.

Head Fixation System and Radiosurgical Procedure

The atraumatic, non-invasive and reproducible Greitz-Bergström head fixation system [2] adapted to

Table 1. *The 1984–1993 Tumour Series Treated at the Centro di Radiochirurgia in Rome*

Tumour type	Patients no.	%
High grade gliomas	498	32%
Low grade gliomas	157	10%
Single metastases	139	9%
Multiple metastases	170	11%
Primary neuro-ectodermal tumours	34	2%
Meningiomas	218	14%
Craniopharyngiomas	35	2%
Pituitary adenomas	85	5%
Acoustic neurinomas	27	2%
Misc.	11	8%
AVMs	78	5%
Total	1560	

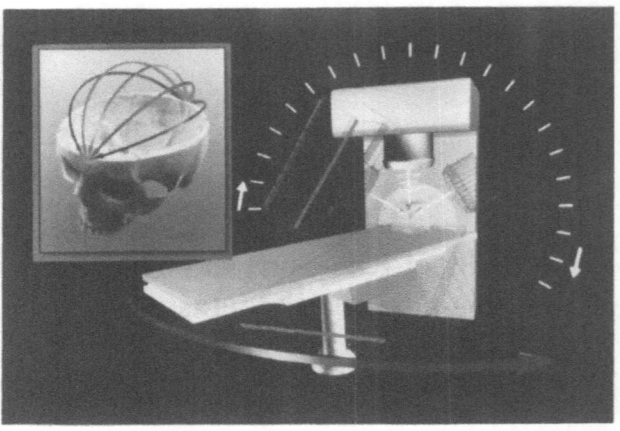

Fig. 2. Linear accelerator stereotactic irradiation is performed through multiple sagittal arches, which are changed whenever radiosurgery is repeated. Compared with 201 Coblat-60 fixed sources of gamma-knife, the rotating linear accelerator beam is focused on the target as if originating, theoretically, from innumerable sources and minimizes radiation to the whole brain

the Fixster frame was used for both the determination of the co-ordinates in CT/NMR scanning and stereotactic irradiation (Fig. 1). The plastic fibre helmet, individually modelled around the head, provided complete fixation enabling the exact transfer of positions between the neuro-radiological and therapeutic procedures. The system was utilized in subsequent CT/NMR staging to obtain strictly comparable neuro-imaging, and tumour response was therefore evaluated precisely and radiosurgery repeated as needed. Neither anaesthesia nor hospitalization of the patient was necessary. Irradiation was performed with a Philips 6 MeV linear accelerator through multiple sagittal arches, using a circular collimator of 10–25 mm according to the size of the target. The angle was varied when radiosurgery was repeated thus reducing radiation to the healthy brain (Fig. 2). The number and width of the arches depended on the tumour size, morphology and location as well as on the prescribed dose, and any variation to the arches allows a different configuration of the isodose.

In metastases not exceeding 25 mm, a 30 Gy single dose was considered effective. The maximum 25 mm collimator was used even for larger metastases as long as the tumour periphery was covered by at least 20 Gy (Fig. 3). When this could not be done we used more than one target depending upon tumour size and configuration. Focusing upon single or multiple targets was facilitated by the 3-D stereotactic NMR, which was the optimal neuro-imaging technique especially for large tumours (Fig. 4).

Follow-up CT/NMR enhanced studies were performed routinely one month after radiosurgery, using the same stereotactic device. If the comparative neuro-imaging showed an unsatisfactory tumour response, radiosurgery was repeated (10–15 Gy additional single dose) soon afterwards at the same session (Fig. 5). The

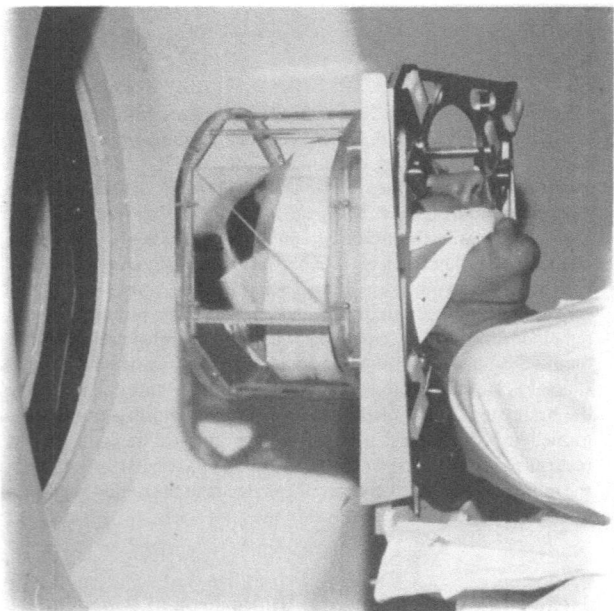

Fig. 1. The non-traumatic Greitz-Bergström pl;astic fibre helmet provides complete head fixation. The individually modelled system is utilized in subsequent CT/NMR staged sittings and re-irradiation, as needed

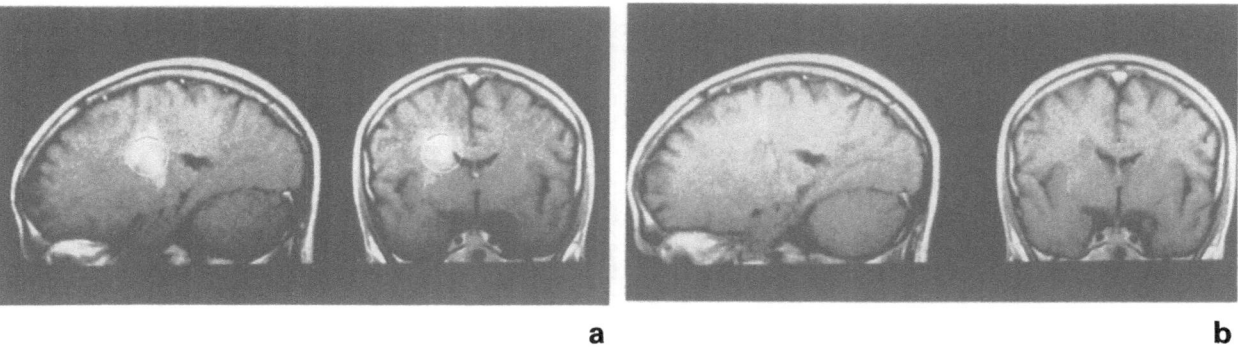

Fig. 3. (a) Single brain metastasis. The target dose for this patient was increased to 40 Gy, to cover the tumour exceeding the 25 mm target with at least 20 Gy. (b) Comparable stereotactic NMR neuro-imaging at 1-month follow-up showed tumour shrinkage

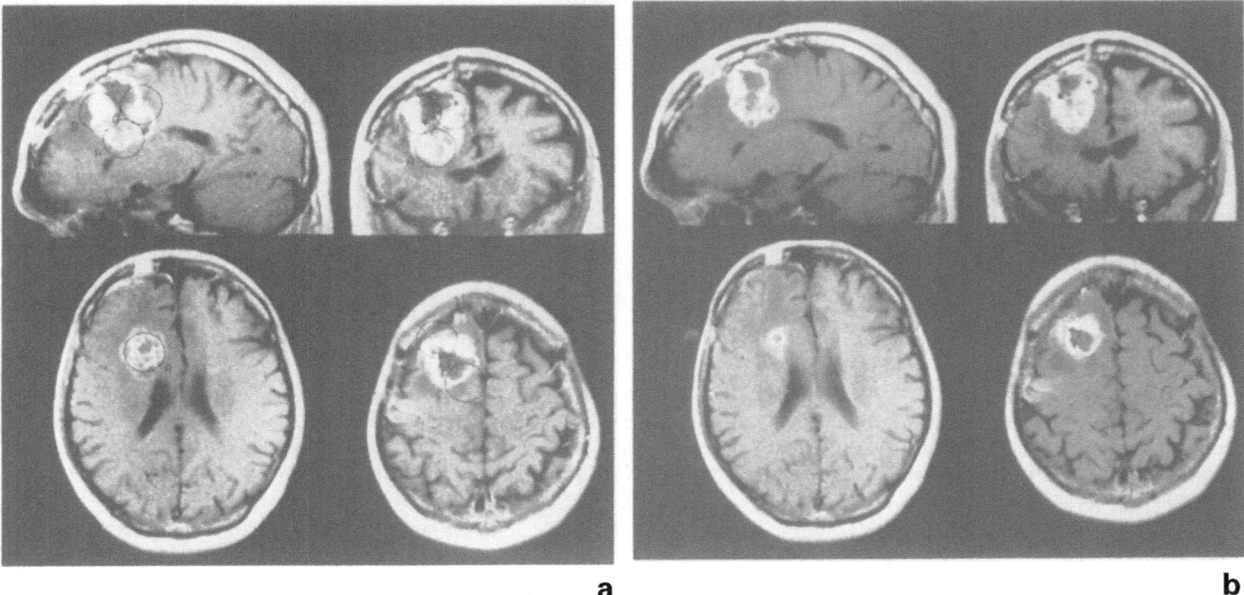

Fig. 4. (a) Recurrent single brain metastasis after 2 operations and conventional radiotherapy. Selected distribution of the three 25 mm targets (A, B, C) detected by 3-D NMR. (b) Comparable stereotactic NMR neuro-imaging at 1-month follow-up showed tumour shrinkage

median total total tumour dose was 50 Gy, ranging from 15 to 80 Gy.

Tumour Response and Results

Results after one single sitting were compared with those obtained after staged sittings (Table 2). A routine follow-up CT/NMR study performed one month after a single radiosurgical sitting revealed the disappearance of the metastasis with resolution of the oedema and mid-line shift in 29 patients (21%). In 85 patients (61%) there was tumour shrinkage with regression of the oedema and decreased pressure on the ventricles.

In 14 patients (10%) the tumour remained unchanged, while in 11 patients (8%) there was tumour progression. Repeat radiosurgery (staged sittings) resulted in complete disappearance of the metastasis in an additional 19 patients (17 with previous shrinkage and 2 with previously unchanged tumour volume). In 33 of the 85 patients with tumour shrinkage, there was further regression of tumour volume, and 8 patients with previously unchanged tumour volume showed tumour shrinkage. The tumour remained refractory to radiosurgery in the 11 patients showing progression of the metastasis at a 1-month follow up. Radiosurgery to a different target (new tumour) was given instantly at

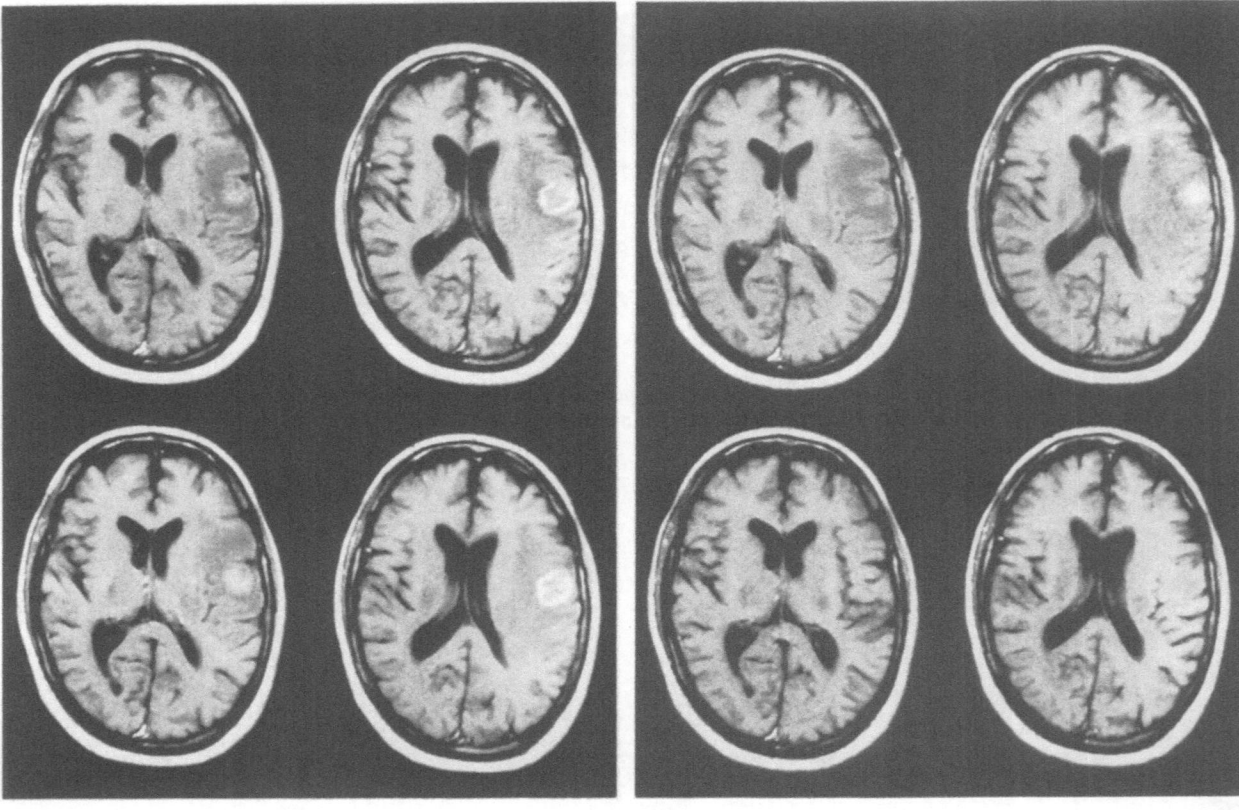

Fig. 5. (a) Upper: Single brain metastasis before Radiosurgery (RS) (30 Gy single dose). Lower: Comparable stereotactic NMR neuro-imaging at 1-month follow-up showed unchanged tumour and oedema. RS was repeated with 15 Gy single dose. (b) Upper: One month after repeat RS comparable stereotactic NMR neuro-imaging showed tumour regression, but with persisting oedema. At the same sitting, RS was again repeated with 10 Gy single dose. Lower: Comparable stereotactic NMR neuro-imaging 1 month later showed complete regression of the tumour and oedema

Table 2. *CT/NMR Tumour Response of Single Cerebral Metastases After Single and 1 or More Repeat Radiosurgical Sittings*

Results	Single sitting	Staged sittings
Tumour disappearance	29 patients (21%)	48 patients (35%)
Tumour shrinkage	85 patients (61%)	76 patients (55%)[a]
Unchanged tumour appearance	14 patients (10%)	4 patients (3%)[b]
Tumour progression	11 patients (8%)	11 patients (8%)

[a] In 17 of the 85 patients there was tumour disappearance and in 33 further shrinkage.

[b] In 2 of the 14 patients there was tumour disappearance and in 8 shrinkage.

a 1-month (or later) CT/NMR follow-up in 22 patients (16%).

The 2-year actuarial survival rate was 12%. The actuarial median survival was 54 weeks for patients treated with radiosurgery alone, and 74 weeks for the 20 patients who underwent radiosurgery after surgical excision of the tumour. A comparison between these data cannot be made, however, as only the more favourable cases are selected for surgery of cerebral metastases.

Discussion and Conclusions

The radiosurgical management we adopt derives from the following considerations:
1. The tumour response, the effect on the oedema and the shifts caused by the metastasis varies from one patient to another, and can be insufficient;
2. metastatic regrowth after initial arrest or regression is expected;
3. the appearance of another brain metastasis at a different site is possible (Fig. 6).

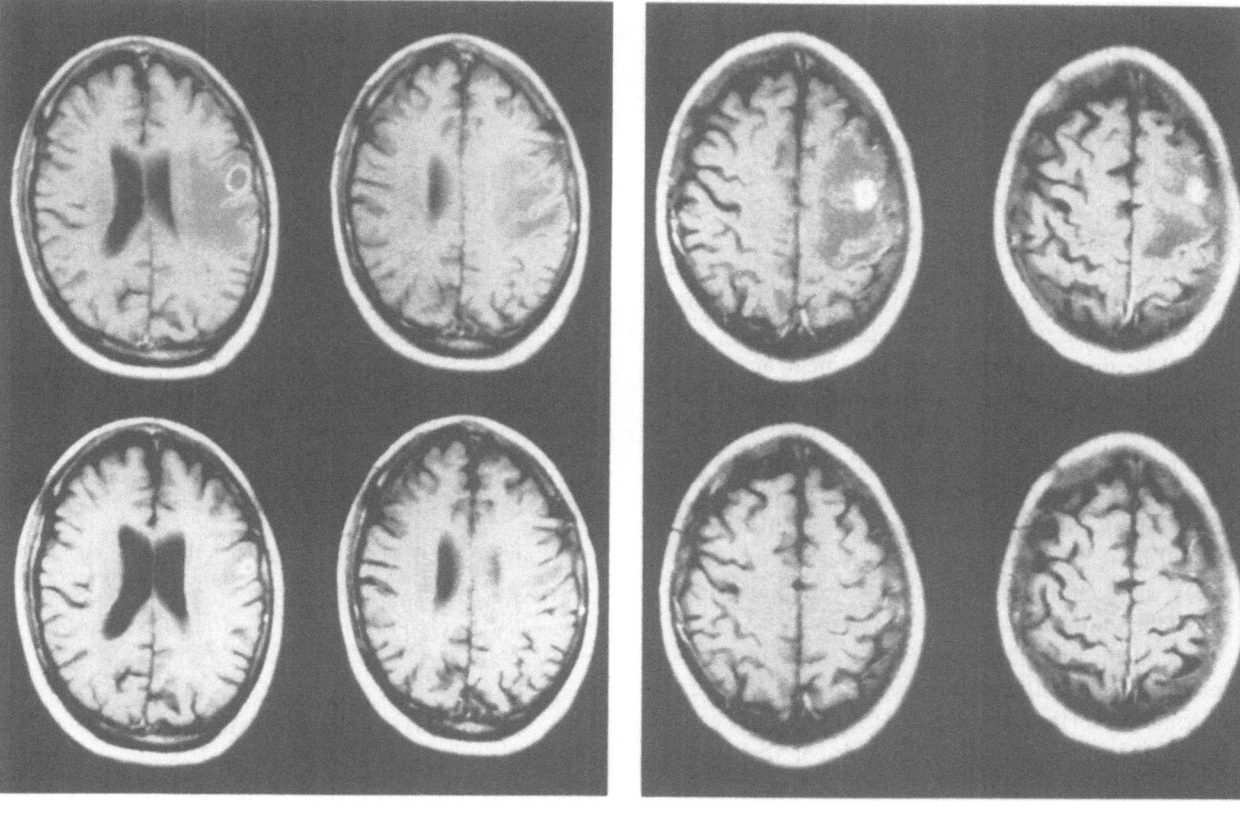

a   **b**

Fig. 6. (a) Upper: Single brain metastasis before RS (30 Gy single dose). Lower: Comparable stereotactic NMR neuro-imaging at 1-month follow-up showed tumour regression and resolution of the oedema. RS was not repeated. (b) Upper: Same patient, same sitting. At a higher level, a new tumour was detected and RS performed with 30 Gy single dose. As non-invasive RS is not time-consuming and hospitalization is not needed, the patient could go home after a couple of hours. Lower: Comparable stereotactic NMR neuro-imaging 1-month later showed tumour disappearance and resolution of the oedema.

In such cases radiosurgery repeated as soon as possible prolongs the comfort and survival of the patient. The technical management undoubtedly depends on the precise evaluation of tumour response, which can only be obtained by strictly comparable neuro-imaging performed with the same initial stereotactic procedure. Therefore, the keystone lies in the non-invasive head fixation system. It allows CT/NMR staging and immediate repeat radiosurgery (if necessary) straight after the diagnostic phase at the same session, without hospitalization, anaesthesia or traumatizing screws into scalp and skull. This simple and time-conserving technique helps and encourages the patient to continue treatment and not give up. Radiosurgery of single brain metastases was first performed in Rome in 1984 (see Valentino [6, 7]) with a single dose of 50 Gy; as there were no guiding references in the literature it was only possible to follow some criteria set out for conventional fractionated radiotherapy. The disappearance of the

metastases led us to experiment with gradually lower radiation doses, until reaching a standardization of results with a dose of 30 Gy as long as the metastasis was entirely within a 25 mm target area. Nevertheless, this dose does fluctuate (higher and lower) depending on the size and site of the metastasis, the radiosensitivity retained by the primary tumour, and the age and clinical condition of the patient.

The 25 mm target is the largest we can use – a conviction reached through experience. Up to the time when we began the routine use of radiosurgery for brain tumours, there had only been sporadic experiences with protons (Kjellberg and Kliman [3]) and the Cobalt-60 gamma-unit (Leksell [4], Norén [5], Backlund [1]) in which the cross-section of each individual beam was 8–14 mm. By using the linear accelerator we tried to gradually increase the size of a special cylindric collimator (through which the thin beam of radiation passed) to 15, 20, 25, 30 mm. The single direct dose to the 30 mm target caused acute reactions (transitory) which induced us to return to a maximum diameter of 25 mm, *versus* the 18 mm then adopted from the gamma-knife [(senseless denomination of the gamma-unit)]. For tumours much larger than 25 mm we use two or more targets to which single doses are directed during the same session.

The results of radiosurgery are influenced by the technical procedure and not by the radiation source, although theoretically, the radiobiological effect should be greater when using the linear accelerator. Cobalt-60 is a radioactive isotope, and due to its progressive decay, more and more time is needed to administer the same dose. The shorter the dose administration time, the greater the radiation efficacy – a factor which could be detrimental to the efficacy of the Cobalt-60 technique. I presume this is the reason why today the techniques using this isotope have universally fallen into disuse.

In conclusion, with our method radiosurgery succeeded in 86% of the 139 patients treated. The disappearance or further shrinkage of the metastasis was the result of the staged sitting in 47% of the patients, without causing any discomfort, not even to the most serious cases. This fact in itself represents a most important ethical aspect which should be considered.

References

1. Backlund EO (1979) Stereotactic radiosurgery in intracranial tumours and vascular malformation In: Advances and technical standards in neurosurgery, Vol 6. Springer, Wien New York
2. Greitz T, Bergström M, Kingsley D *et al* (1980) Head fixation system for integration of radiodiagnostic and therapeutic procedures. Neuroradiology 19: 1–6
3. Kjellberg RN, Kliman B (1973) A-system for therapy of pituitary tumours. In: Kohler PO, Ross Gt (eds.) Diagnosis and treatment of pituitary tumours. Excerpta Medica, Amsterdam
4. Leksell L (1971) Stereotaxis and radiosurgery an operative system. Thomas, Springfield
5. Norén G, Arndt J, Hindmarsh (1983) Stereotactic radiosurgery in cases of acoustic neurinoma: further experiences. Neurosurgery 13: 12–22
6. Valentino V (1986) Stereotactic radiation therapy in arterio-venous malformations and brain tumours using Fixter system. Acta Radiol (Stockholm) 369 [Suppl]: 215–219
7. Valentino V (1988) Radiosurgery in cerebral tumors and AVM Acta Neurochir (Wien) [Suppl] 42: 139–197

Correspondence: Vincenzo Valentino, M. D., Centro di Radiochirurgia, Clinica Flaminia, Via Luigi Bodio 5B, I-00191 Roma, Italy.

Acta Neurochir (1995) [Suppl] 63: 101–108

Malignant Transformation of Benign Gliomas During Interstitial Irradiation

D. Hellwig[1], H. D. Mennel[2], B. L. Bauer[1], E. List-Hellwig[3], E. A. Koop[1], and H. O. Neidel[4]

[1]Department of Neurosurgery, [2]Department of Neuropathology, [3]Department of Radiology, and [4]Department of Radiotherapy, Philipps University Marburg, Federal Republic of Germany

Summary

Interstitial curietherapy with 125-Iodine is an effective therapeutic option in the treatment of low grade gliomas. Four cases with astrocytoma grade II are presented, where tumour growth characteristics have changed to anaplasia during interstitial irradiation after a primary period of tumour regression.

Anaplastic transformation could be due to a radiation effect or an insufficient therapeutic influence of interstitial irradiation on natural tumour progression of glioma growth due to genetic events.

Keywords: Glioma; stereotactic neurosurgery; interstitial irradiation; anaplastic transformation; neuroendoscopy.

Introduction

Different views are held concerning spontaneous and induced malignant transformation in gliomas. The concept of increasing morphological pleomorphism of cells and tissue in supratentorial gliomas of adults is based on the assumption that there is progression in malignancy between isomorphic astrocytoma to anaplastic astrocytoma and glioblastoma multiforme. Results of molecular biology strongly support this view, which on the other hand forms the basis of intracranial tumour grading.

In contrast, papers reporting malignant transformation of formerly low grade gliomas after and due to therapy strategies of different kind have appeared. Lately, an increase of second malignancies unrelated to the primary tumour has been supposed. Most of the reported transformations and secondaries concern external irradiation and chemotherapy. We report here a few cases of rapid malignant development after interstitial irradiation of low grade gliomas.

Methods and Patients

Operative Technique and Instrumentation

In general stereotactic operations were performed under local anaesthesia with slight sedation. In children and for operations in the posterior fossa general anaesthesia was used.

We used the CT-compatible instrumentation of Mundinger and Birg [17]. The target point calculation was carried out with the computer-program TARGETRM (Fischer MET, Freiburg). In some special cases stereotactic biopsies were done under endoscopic control.

Histopathological Examination

Morphological diagnosis was performed intra-operatively by smear preparation technique or postoperatively by conventional histopathological examination. Tissue specimens were obtained in mm steps from the marginal areas to the center going on to the distal border of the lesion. In this way we got an overview about the histopathological structure as a whole especially about the homogeneity of the glioma.

With the method of intra-operative smear preparation special caution is required in evaluating diagnostic reliability. Our diagnostic security increased since 1980 from 70% to 90% correct diagnoses today, both for tumour entity and grade [16]. Yet, this diagnostic reliability largely reposes on serial studies of 550 tumour specimens obtained by open surgery, analyzed by smear preparation and subsequent conventional methods.

Interstitial Curietherapy

Interstitial curietherapy for therapy of low grade gliomas was performed with permanent application of 125-Iodine seeds. Dosimetry was calculated with a special three-dimensional program using the EVADOS system (Siemens Inc.). The peripheral tumour dose was fixed at about 75 Gy. 125-Iodine seed application was performed with the seed application set of Fischer MET, Freiburg.

Patient's Selection and Follow-up

Interstitial curietherapy with permanent 125-Iodine seed application was carried out in patients with low grade gliomas, not only in the cerebral midline but also for tumours in so-called "eloquent" brain regions. The patients were discharged from the hospital six days after intervention. Long-term follow-up was done by regular clinical and CT control examinations.

Case Reports

Case 1

A 40 year old woman was admitted in December 1983 after onset of focal seizures. Computed tomography demonstrated a large right temporal tumour, which was completely removed by open surgery. Histopathological examination revealed a low grade glioma: Fibrillary astrocytes formed a loose network with numerous small cysts. Special stains for glial fibers and immunohistochemistry entirely confirmed the diagnosis of fibrillary astrocytoma.

The subsequent clinical course was unremarkable. CT controls during the first three years consistently documented no tumour recurrence. In April 1988, however, a large recurrence was noted by imaging methods, which were performed after the onset of headache and vomiting. The recurrent tumour was now approached stereotactically; again a low grade astrocytoma was diagnosed in several probes removed. Interstitial curietherapy was performed with permanent application of three 125-Iodine seeds. Seven months later a mass shifting of the midline caused by the perifocal oedema, and a space occupying cystic lesion occured. Yet the patient was in good neurological and physical condition during this time and during the following three years. Several CT control examinations excluded remaining or recurrent tumour growth.

In September 1991 the patient suffered anew from headache and vomiting and additional visual disturbances. This time the CT scan documented a contrast enhancing tumour with midline shift. The tumour was now approached by open surgery; its final diagnosis was that of a glioblastoma multiforme. Nine months later and nine years after onset of symptoms and first intervention the patient died. No postmortem examination was performed (Fig. 1a–d, Fig. 2a–d).

Case 2

A 25 year old man underwent CT analysis after a first grand meal seizure. A small hypodense lesion was localized in the right temporal lobe. The stereotac-

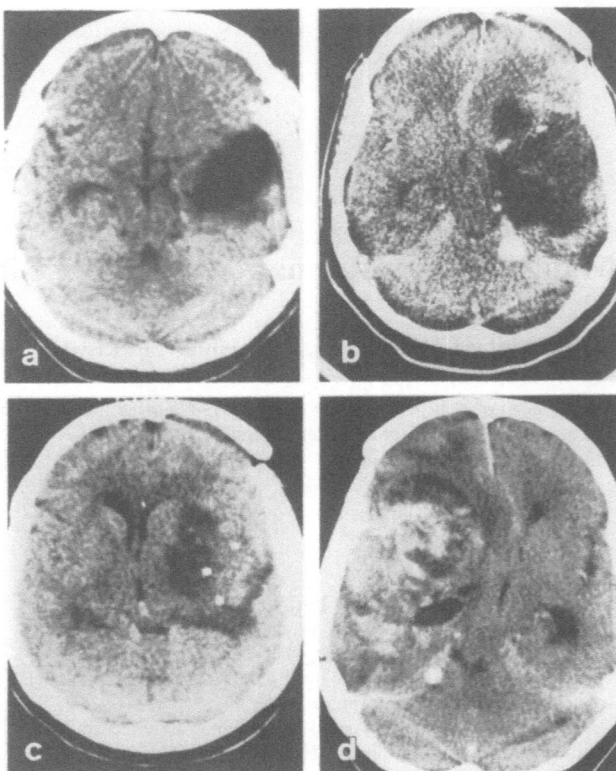

Fig. 1. CT scans of case 1. (a) Right temporal predominantly hypodense lesion in December 1983 diagnosed as astrocytoma grade II. (b) Recurrent tumour with mass displacement and increased tumour volume in April 1988 diagnosed again as astrocytoma grade II. (c) Tumour after seed implantation in June 1988. (d) CT-scan of second recurrence in June 1992 presenting as malignant glioma. (Note change of hemispheric lateralization in CT technique)

tically removed tissue in five different probes showed fibrillary astrocytes without signs of pleomorphism or mitotic activity. The diagnosis was fibrillary astrocytoma (WHO) grade II. Interstitial irradiation by implantation of a single 125-Iodine seed with an accumulation dose of 75 Gy was performed. Nine months later, CT control revealed oedema and lateral displacement of the right hemisphere and a small rim with contrast enhancement surrounding the implanted seed. Renewed CT control after five more months displayed no more signs of remaining or recurrent tumour. The patient felt well until May 1992.

At this time the patient began to suffer from headache and loss of concentration, but neurological symptoms were absent. Now a large cystic neoplasm next to the site of the primary tumour was detected. After tumour resection the final diagnosis of glioblastoma multiforme was established (Fig. 3a–d, Fig. 4a and b).

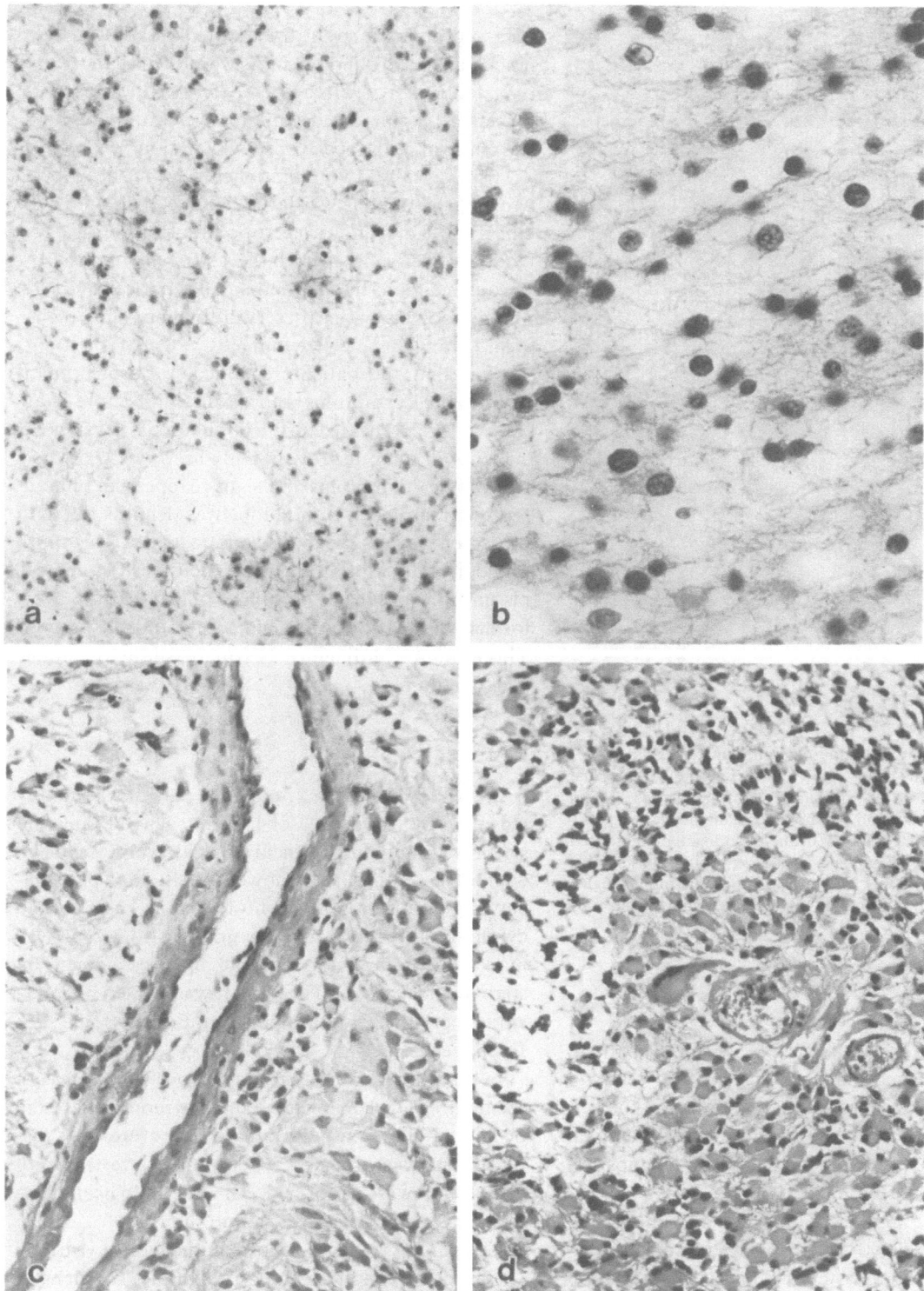

Fig. 2. Malignant transformation of formerly low grade astrocytoma in case 1. (a) Loose network of primary astrocytoma. In the lower part formation of larger cyst. Many glial processes are visible. GFAP, x 125. (b) Higher magnification of low grade astrocytoma in case 1. Loose network of processes and microcystic degeneration is documented by status spongiosus. Cresyl violet, x 500. (c) After malignant transformation, pronounced perivascular arrangement of huge astrocytes occurs, HE x 250. (d) Marked cellular pleomorphism with perivascular arrangement of gemistocytic astrocytes, giant cells and in the upper part of the picture small round cells, HE x 205

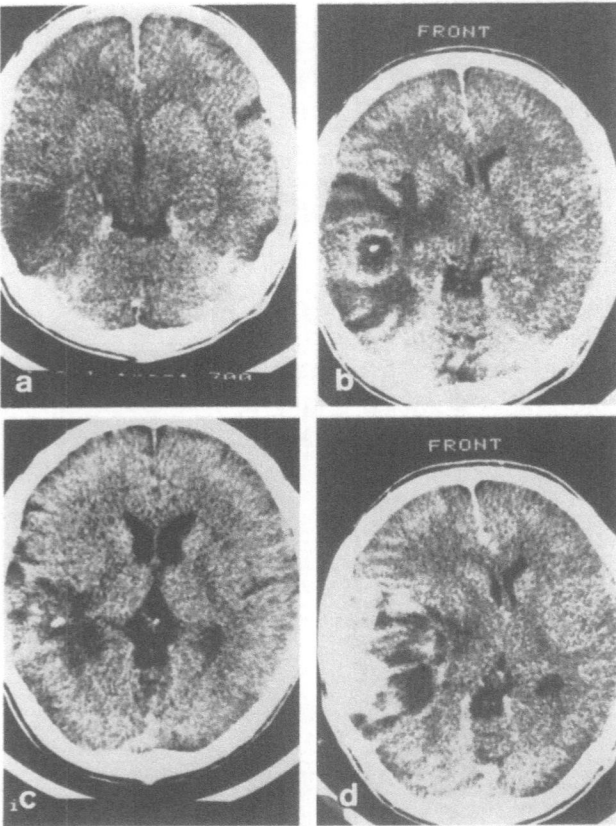

Fig. 3. CT pictures during tumour evolution in case 2. (a) Hypo-dense lesion without mass displacement in July 1990. His-topathological diagnosis was fibrillary astrocytoma grade II. (b) Enhancement of a rim around the implanted radio-active seed in CT control examination in March 1991 due to an irradiation induced disturbance of blood brain barrier disruption. (c) Considerable regression of tumour volume after interstitial irradiation in August 1991. (d) Regrowth of transformed glioblastoma with considerable midline shift in May 1992

Case 3

This case dates back to April 1987, when the patient, a 34 year old woman had her first seizure. CT-scan depicted a space occupying hypodensity in the left frontal lobe. Stereotactic biopsy with stepwise removal of several minute tissue probes led to the diagnosis of benign astrocytoma.

Renewed cytological diagnosis and interstitial curietherapy were performed in an external depart-ment of functional and stereotactic neurosurgery re-nowned for its long experience in this field.

Morphological diagnosis was confirmed as proto-plasmatic astrocytoma. The therapy applied a total activity of 17.6 mCi and an accumulating dose of 75 Gy. During the first months after seed implantation

a series of epileptic seizures was noted. In January 1988 much oedema around the seeds was noted as the cause of epileptic activity. In September 1988, the mass dis-placement required a decompressive craniotomy and the removal of the space occupying lesion.

Histologically two components were described. Most of the tumour was large radionecrosis with cal-cification, amorphous necrotic transformation, oc-cluded vessels and inert large astrocytes as well as fibrous reaction. In a second smaller part, protoplas-mic astrocytoma was preserved, but no signs of in-creased malignancy were found.

After that the patient remained free from major neurological symptoms and seizures for more than three years. Repeated CT examinations never gave evidence of tumour growth. Only in May 1992, when neurological symptoms and signs reappeared, tumour regrowth in the left frontal lobe was demonstrated. It presented as a large partly cystic mass. The mor-phological description this time mentions cytological pleomorphism such as occurence of giant cells, newly-formed vasculature and even necrotic transformation. This tumour was diagnosed as anaplastic astrocytoma (Fig. 5a and b).

Case 4

In November 1987 a 27 old male patient was admit-ted after the occurence of his first general epileptic seizure without further neurological symptoms. The computed tomography showed a left side space oc-cupying lesion in the frontotemporal region. The cytological diagnosis of a low grade astrocytoma was made by examination of four biopsies gained by stereotactic removal. The patient was treated by inter-stitial curietherapy with implantation of four 125-Iodine seeds.

In the following months the space occupying effect of the perifocal oedema increased. Nine months after the beginning of interstitial irradiation a severe mass dis-placement was observed. A decompressive temporal lobectomy was performed. Histopathological diag-nosis revealed mild gliosis but no tumour.

The patient was then followed up over five years; he was in good condition during this time. No signs of tumour regrowth were observed until 1993, almost exactly six years after the onset of the first symptoms. The CT scan now presented new tumour growth documented by contrast enhancing areas as well as volume increase with unilateral ventricular compres-

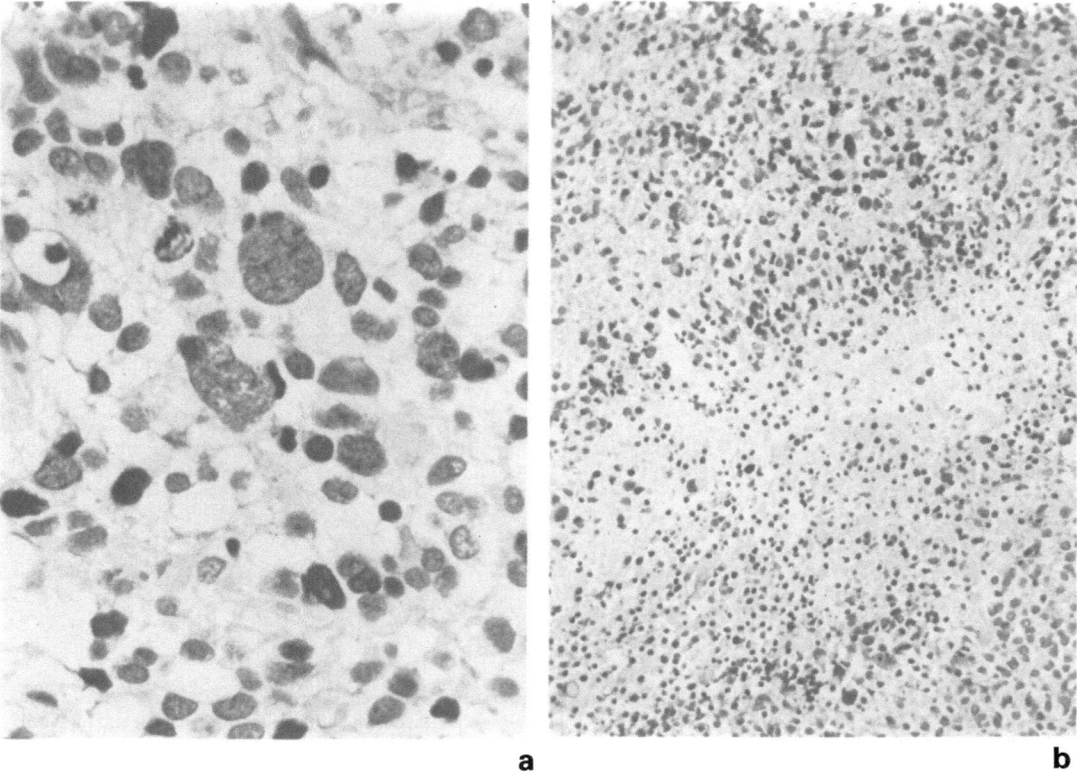

Fig. 4. Malignant transformation of formerly low grade astrocytoma in case 2. (a) Cellular pleomorphism and occurrence of giant cells, small round cells and single necroses in glioblastoma multiforme. Cresyl violet, x 500. (b) Small elongated necrosis with formation of pseudopalisades documents architectural polymorphism. Cresyl violet, × 250

sion and mass shift. These findings were interpreted as tumour recurrence and increase in malignancy (Fig. 6a–d).

Discussion

We present here four cases of low grade gliomas treated by interstitial irradiation successfully over the years, which recurred as gliomas of a higher malignancy. Two developments have taken place recently, which make it feasible to discuss the possibilities of natural or induced malignant transformation of formerly benign gliomas:

First: Evidence is strongly accumulating that in supratentorial gliomas of the adult there is a natural tumour progression due to genetic events.
Second: Differentiated therapeutic strategies were developed for a variety of lesions, which obviously lead to prolonged survival.

Natural tumour progression in human supratentorial gliomas in the adult has been held as a possibility for some time. H. J. Scherer in 1940 had coined the denomination "primary glioblastoma" that was considered to develop de novo as opposed to secondary glioblastoma thought to be transformed from pre-existing benign glioma [22]. Natural progression in supratentorial gliomas as a concept equally underlies the grading system adopted by Zülch and Wechsler [27]. Different grades of gliomas are described morphologically by stepwise increase of pleomorphism of the cell and tissue level [15].

In the meantime, the term "glioma progression" has gained a clearcut significance also in terms of molecular biology and genetics [12]. Furthermore, a concept explaining the malignancy progression by enhanced but nevertheless insufficient angiogenesis emerges [20]. Thus it seems reasonable to admit that low grade astrocytomas have the potential to transform into malignant forms; such a transformation has been described repeatedly [23, 24]. Yet, there is considerable insecurity in discrimination of the two forms by morphological analysis alone, if one is completely sure that secondary malignant development occurred, checked

106   D. Hellwig *et al.*: Malignant Transformation of Benign Gliomas

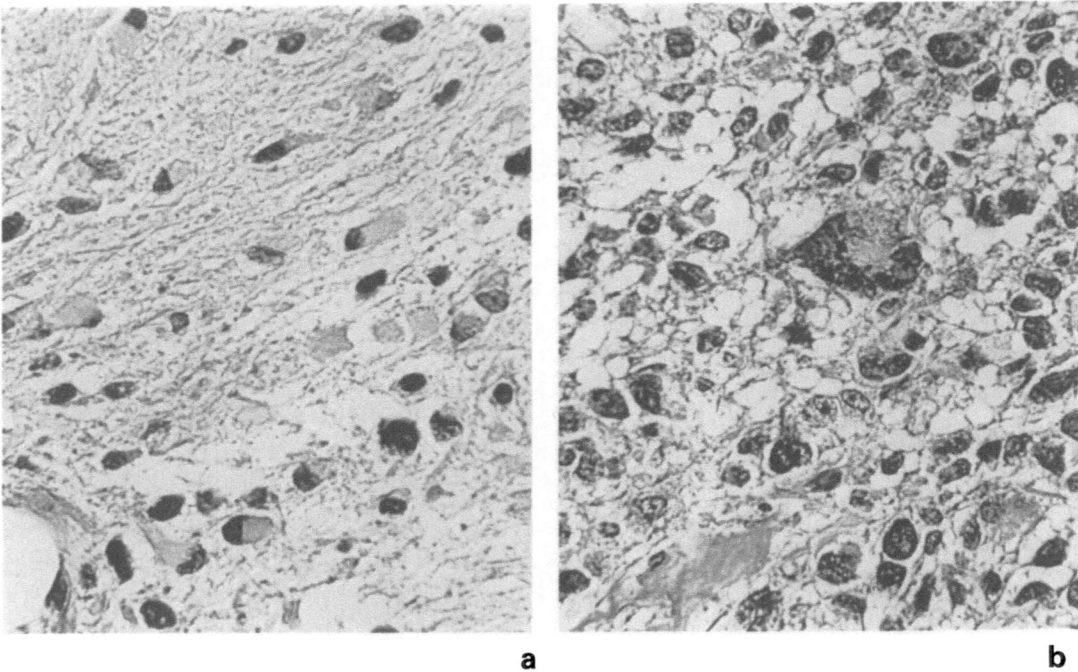

a   b

Fig. 5. Histopathologic appearance of low grade glioma (II) and malignant transformation (III) in case 3. (a) Assembly of large gemistocytic cells in low to moderate density in a thoroughly fibrillary matrix. HE, x 500. (b) Cellular pleomorphism with giant cell formation and high cell density in the transformed anaplastic astrocytoma. HE, × 500

by two complete tumour analyses after a due interval. The latter condition however is restricted to a few cases as in our report and probably most of them are gained after (and possibly because of) effective treatment.

The possibilities of more differentiated treatment schedules — as the second point — are obviously more effective, even if the pertinent statistics document increases in lifespan to a limited extent only. But large studies have been performed [4, 5, 13] that in a simplified summary had two main results:

Firstly: in the outcome of treated malignant gliomas, there are about 20% of tumour bearers who take advantage from the protocols and secondly: predictive factors have emerged that may give an indication which patients profit from a given protocol and which do not.

In addition, surgical techniques in recent years have become increasingly more sophisticated and efficient. The indications for interstitial irradiation have been enlarged and refined [18, 19, 25]. The endoscopic approach is increasingly used and allows a removal of probes for diagnosis in relevant areas promising to reduce tissue damage to true "minimal invasion" [1, 7, 8].

Thus we deal with an evolution which may produce the time course necessary for the manifestation of secondary malignancies. On the other hand, the causative role of irradiation in any kind of tumour formation and progress in gliomas in animals has been restricted to single cases [11], but few authors admitted a causative relationship between irradiation and malignant glioma formation in monkeys [6].

As to human cases, the various intracranial tumours reported to occur after irradiation are listed in some textbooks of neuro-oncology [9, 10]. A minority of them only are true malignant gliomas [14, 21]. Thus, irradiation as a cause of malignant evolution in tumours of the glioma group has been considered reluctantly. Therefore, the malignant transformation in four of our treated cases during the last years seems noteworthy. For the time being, the possible causative role of the interstitial irradiation must remain open. The nowdays affirmed "natural" progression of low grade into high grade astrocytomas together with effective treatment – as documented in our cases, may suffice as an explanation for the malignant conversion of formerly benign tumours.

Yet there is a second point, which has to be considered. In two of our cases there was increased intracranial

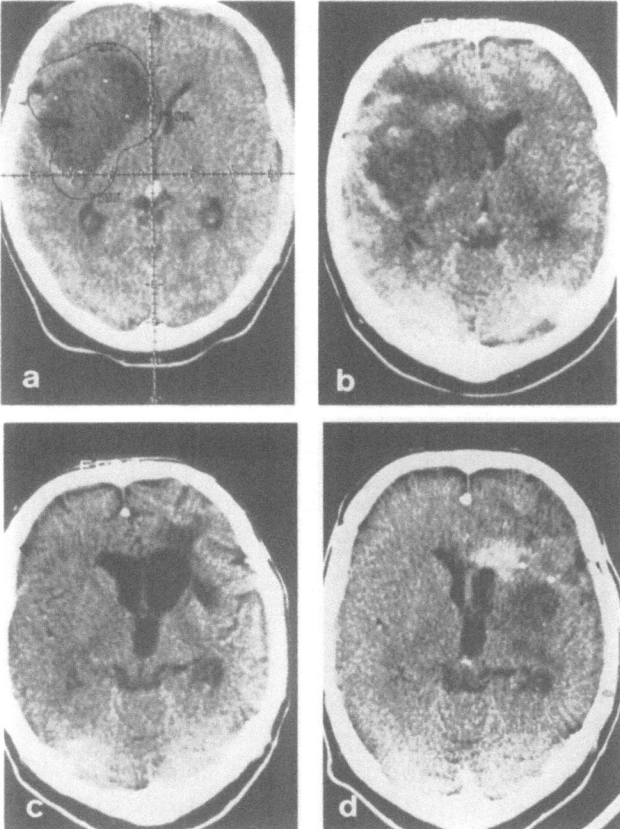

Fig. 6. Tumour development in case 4. (a) The left sided space occupying hypodense lesion was detected in November 1987. The CT picture is shown with the volumetric calculation for interstitial irradiation. (b) In June 1992, severe mass displacement required a decompressive partial temporal lobectomy. (c) In December 1990, no tumour was present. As a consequence of interstitial irradiation the anterior horn of the left lateral ventricle was enlarged. (Note change in hemispheric lateralization in CT technique). (d) CT control in December 1993, six years after diagnosis of a low grade glioma, showed a contrast enhancing tumour recurrence with compression of the left anterior horn. Growth characteristics of this space occupying lesion are suspicious of the development of a malignant glioma

pressure during effective therapy obviously not due to tumour regrowth, this mass effect is wellknown and described elsewhere [26]. This is documented in Fig. 3b by an enhancing rim around the central seed and voluminous perifocal oedema. In the CT examination such a circular formation around the radiation source is rather indicative of resorptive events than of newformed tumour. It is almost impossible to discriminate reactive changes due to effective therapy from overt tumour growth by imaging methods. As shown here, even mass displacement is no reliable indicator. In case 4, mass displacement lead to temporal lobe

resection which was followed by good clinical improvement of the patient for a number of years.

References

1. Bauer BL, Hellwig D (1994) Intracranial and intraspinal endoscopy. Minimally invasive endoscopic neurosurgery. In: Schmidek HH, Sweet WH (eds) Operative neurosurgical techniques, 3rd Ed. Saunders, Philadelphia, in press
2. David E, Unger RR (1967) Zur Problematik maligne entarteter Gliome des Großhirns Teil I. Arch Geschwulstforsch 29: 331–354
3. David E, Unger RR (1967) Zur Problematik maligne entarteter Gliome des Großhirns, Teil II. Arch Geschwulstforsch 30: 135–141
4. EORTC Brain Tumor Group (1978) Effect of CCNU on survival rate of objective remission and duration of free interval in patients with malignant gliomas – final evaluation. Eur J Cancer 14: 851–856
5. European Organization for Research on Treatment of Cancer (EORTC) Brain Tumor Group (1981) Evaluation of CCNU, VM 26 plus CCNU and procarbazine in supratentorial brain gliomas. Final evaluation of a randomized study. J Neurosurg 55: 27–31
6. Haymaker W, Rubinstein LJ, Miquel J (1972) Brain tumours in irradiated monkeys. Acta Neuropat 20: 267–277
7. Hellwig D, Bauer BL (1992) Minimally invasive neurosurgery by means of ultrathin endoscopes. Acta Neuroch (Wien) [Suppl] 54: 63–68
8. Hellwig D, Bauer BL (1993) Diagnostik und Therapie intrakranieller Tumoren. TW Neurologie Psychiatrie 7: 347–356
9. Jänisch W, Güthert H, Schreiber D (1976) Pathologie der Tumoren des Zentralnervensystems. Fischer, Jena
10. Jänisch W, Schreiber D, Güthert H (1988) Neuropathologie: Tumoren des Nervensystems. Gustav Fischer, Stuttgart
11. Kent SP, Pickering JE (1958) Neoplasms in monkey (Macaca mulatta) spontaneous and irradiation induced. Cancer 11: 138–147
12. Kleihues P, Burger PC, Scheithauer BW (1993) The new WHO classification of brain tumours. Brain Pathol 3: 255–268
13. Krauseneck P, Mertens HP (1987) Results of chemotherapy of malignant brain tumours in adults. In: Jellinger K (ed) Therapy of malignant brain tumours. Springer, Wien New York
14. Marus G, Levin CV, Rutherford GS (1986) Malignant glioma following radiotherapy for unrelated primary tumours. Cancer 58: 886–894
15. Mennel HD, Plate KH (1991) Morphologie und Prognose bei intrakraniellen Tumoren. Fortschr Neurol Psychiat 59: 35–68
16. Mennel HD, Hellwig D, Bauer BL (1994) Ergebnisse und Zuverlässigkeit stereotaktisch und endoskopisch gewonnener Probebiopsate bei Hirntumoren. Zentrbl Neurochir 55: 79–91
17. Mundinger F, Birg W (1984) Stereotactic biopsy of intracranial processes. Acta Neurochir (Wien) Suppl 33: 219–224
18. Mundinger F, Weigel K (1988) Considerations in the usage and results of curietherapy. In: Lunsford LD (ed) Modern stereotactic neurosurgery. Martinus Nijhoff, Boston, pp: 245–258
19. Ostertag CB, Warnke PC (1987) Brachytherapy of gliomas. J Neurooncol 5: 179
20. Plate KH, Breier G, Weich HA, Risau W (1992) Vascular endothelial growth factor is a potential tumorangiogenesis factor in human gliomas invivo. Nature 359: 845–848
21. Robinson RG (1978) A second brain tumour and irradiation. J Neurol Neurosurg Psychiatry 41: 1005–1012

22. Scherer HJ (1940) The pathology of cerebral gliomas. J Neurol Psychiatr 3: 147–177
23. Schmitt HP (1983) Rapid anaplastic transformation of gliomas in childhood. Neuropediatrics 14: 137–143
24. Schmitt HP (1983) Rapid anaplastic transformation of gliomas in adulthood. "Selection" in neurooncogenesis. Path Res Pract 176: 313–323
25. Sturm V, Schlegel W, Bauer B, Wowra B, *et al* (1987) Interstitial irradiation of low grade gliomas with 125-I. Treatment panning, possibilities and limitations. J Neurooncol 5: 184
26. Wowra B, Schmitt HP, Sturm V (1989) Incidence of late radiation necrosis with transient mass effect after interstitial low dose rate radiotherapy for cerebral gliomas. Acta Neurochir (Wien) 99: 104–108
27. Zülch KJ, Wechsler W (1968) Pathology and classification of gliomas. Progr Neurol Surg 2: 1–84

Correspondence: Dieter Hellwig, M. D., Neurochirurgische Klinik, Philipps Universität Marburg, Baldingerstrasse, D-35033 Marburg, Federal Republic of Germany.

Acta Neurochir (1995) [Suppl] 63: 109–114

Stereotactic Radiosurgery: The Lyon Experience

F. P. Rocher, I. Sentenac, C. Berger, I. Marquis, P. Romestaing, and **J. P. Gerard**

Service de Radiothérapie et Oncologie, Centre Hospitalier Lyon-Sud, Pierre Bénite, France

Summary

From 10/1989 to 12/1992, 135 patients were treated, in Lyon, by Stereotactic Radiosurgery (RS) +/− External beam Radiotherapy (EBRT). Indications were AVMs or tumours that could not be cured by embolisation or/and surgery and are not larger than 30 to 35 mm. Lesions received 15 to 20 Gy (70% isodose) in one course. Among the 42 AVMs, only one rebled 6 months after RS and 9/15 had clinical improvement. Thirty-one had a radiological follow-up of 4 to 29 months after RS. Ten were totally obliterated, seven regressed more than 80% and six had a reduction of 50 to 80% of their AVM. Three grade 3 radio necrosis occurred for a cerebral trunk AVM and two large lesions. Three of the 15 treated meningiomas progressed after RS, 2 of them were controlled by conventional surgery. Four out of nine presenting symptoms had clinical improvement and, with a radiological follow-up of 4 to 24 months, 5 were stabilised and 6 regressed. Two grade three complications occurred for large lesions. The biological and radiological results of RS were good for the 42 treated pituitary adenomas but the high visual complication rate (12/42 with 8 grade 3) was too important and we stopped RS for these tumours except for small (less than 2 cm) adenoma at some distance from the optic chiasma. The visual complications were related to the tumour volume, the distance between the adenoma and the visual tract and pre-existent visual alterations. The RS dose is now reduced for all lesions larger than 20 mm and a new fractionated technique will be developed to reduce the complication rate and to improve tumour control.

Keywords: Radiosurgery; arteriovenous malformation; meningioma; pituitary adenoma.

Introduction

Stereotactic Radiosurgery is a very elegant non-invasive technique used to treat intracranial lesions without open surgery. Since the first description of this technique in San Francisco in 1945 and the development due to Leksell *et al.* in Sweden since 1949, Radiosurgery (RS) has been extensively developed in many centres. Three major techniques are used: particle beams, gamma-units and modified linacs with equivalent results. We will expose here the first three years of experience of RS in Lyon. We used a linac based technique and we selected our cases with single non surgical lesions accurately delineated which could not have been treated by new embolisation and the largest diameter of which was less than 30 to 35 millimetres.

Methods and Material

We use, in Lyon, a linac-based radiosurgery technique, similar to the technique developed in Boston by Lutz *et al.*, Saunders *et al.* [15, 19] and previously described [16, 20].

Briefly, a Brown-Roberts-Wells stereotactic frame (Radionics) is fixed to the patient's skull under local anaesthesia the morning of the treatment procedure. The lesion co-ordinates are defined by angiography and/or a computed tomography and 3D reconstruction of the lesion is performed with a custom-designed computer system. The patient is placed in the treatment position with the frame fixed to an isocentric table specially designed in our department which places the lesion center on the isocenter of a linac Saturne 20 (GE-CGR MeV). The irradiation is delivered with 18 MV photons through a lead circular collimator of 8 to 30 millimeters in diameter. We have always treated a single isocenter with four arcs (one transverse, one sagittal and two obliques) in a total of 470 to 540 degrees. Fifteen to 20 Gy are delivered on the 70% isodose.

When delivered, the external beam radiotherapy (EBRT) is delivered with 10 or 18 MV photons and 2 to 4 beams adjusted to CT contrast enhanced tumour with a margin of 1 to 2 centimeters. A personal mask insures the immobilisation of the head and also the reproducibility of the treatment. Five fractions of 1.8 to 2 Gy are administered every week for a total dose of 36 to 50.4 Gy.

Between October 1989 and December 1992, we have treated 135 patients aged from 10 to 80 for AVMs, pituitary adenomas, meningiomas and others primary and secondary tumours as reported in Table 1. Arteriovenous malformations were the most frequent treated lesions and concerned 42 patients aged from 10 to 67 (mean 35). The treatment characteristics are summarised in Table 2. According to the Spetzler classification, 11 patients had a grade I–II AVM, 19 were grade III and 12 were grade IV–V. The treatment was only radiosurgery for 19 patients (1 patient received 2 courses of radiosurgery and a second one had received previous radiosurgery in another center). Fifteen lesions were previously embolised, 1 to

Table 1. *Characteristics of the 135 Lesions Treated by Radiosurgery in Lyon Between 10/1989 and 12/1992*

AVM	42	Glioma	5
Pituitary adenoma	36	Pineal tumours	4
Meningioma	15	Chordoma	2
Astrocytoma I–II	13	Craniopharyngioma	2
Neurinoma	8	Nasopharynx	1
Metastases	7		

Table 2. *Treatment Characteristics of the 42 AVMs Treated by Radiosurgery*

Grade (Spetzler)	I–II = 11
	III = 19
	IV = 12
Treatments	RS = 19
	embol + RS = 15
	surgery + RS = 6
	surgery + embol + RS = 2
Collimator (∅)	12.5–17.5 mm = 10
	20–22.5 mm = 5
	25–30 mm = 28
Dose	35 patients = 20 Gy
	5 patients > 20 mm = 15 to 18.75 Gy
	2 patients with 2nd RS = 15 Gy

RS radiosurgery, *embol* embolisation.

3 times before radiosurgery, 6 had surgery and 2 had surgery plus embolisation before radiosurgery (Fig. 1). The 2 previously treated patients received only 15 Gy and 5 patients treated since April 1992 for a residual lesion of more than 20 mm recived 15 to 18.75 Gy (70% isodose) according to their size and location. All of the other patients received 20 Gy. Fifteen patients aged from 33 to 80 years (mean 54) were treated for 7 primary meningiomas and 8 recurrences. Table 3 summarises the characteristics of these tumours and there treatments. They were either recurrent tumours after surgery (plus EBRT

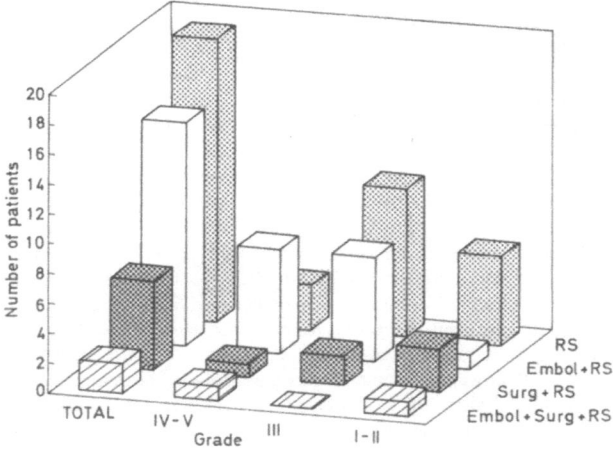

Fig. 1. Treatment modality for the 42 AVMs (Spetzler classification)

for 2) or non-removable ones. Thirty-six pituitary adenomas were treated for patients aged from 23 to 74 (mean 54). All of them were treated either for a residual tumour after surgery or a recurrence. Table 4 summarises the main characteristics of these tumours. About half of them were gonadotropic or non-secreting adenomas and 61% (22/36) were larger than 2 cm. All of them received 20 Gy.

The complications were graded, according to the WHO classification, as grade 1–2 when no treatment or only medical treatment is needed, grade 3 if surgery or hospitalisation is needed, grade 4 if the complication is life threatening and grade 5 in case of death.

Results

AVMs

The mean follow up for the 42 patients treated for an AVM was 14 months (4 to 29 months). Only one patient rebled 6 months after the RS. It was a large unresectable grade IV lesion. When it rebled, partial regression of the AVM allowed embolisation and a complete surgical removal. Upon 15 patients presenting neurological symptoms before RS, 9 had clinical improvement after the treatment. Seven grade 1–2 complications such as headache, transient aphasia or seizures occurred 1 to 13 months after RS (mean 6.6 months). All regressed. Three grade 3 necroses occurred 9, 17 and 19 months after RS. After 16 months of

Table 3. *Characteristics of the 15 Patients Treated by RS for a Meningioma*

Location	8 cavernous sinus – 1 optic nerve
	2 clivus – 1 tentorium cerebelli – 1 occipital
	1 falx cerebri – 1 posterior fossa
Other treatments	surgery = 1 primary (biopsy) + 8 recurrences
	EBRT = 6 concomitant (36 to 50.4 Gy) + 2 previous
Collimator (∅)	15–20 mm = 5
	22.5–25 mm = 5
	30 mm = 5
Dose	12 patients = 20 Gy
	3 patients = 12.5; 15; 15 Gy

Table 4. *Characteristics of the 36 Pituitary Adenomas Treated by RS*

Type	GH = 10 – TSH = 1
	prolactin = 4 – corticotropic = 6
	gonadotropic/non secreting = 15
Collimator (∅)	12.5 – 20 mm = 14
	22.5 – 25 mm = 15
	30 mm = 7
Dose	36 patients = 20 Gy

improvement, one patient with a brainstem AVM had a very poor clinical course with partial necrosis of a main feeding vessel. The other two patients were treated with a 30 mm collimator and received 20 Gy. One had persistent seizures after a cerebral necrosis and the other suffered persistent hemianopsia with headaches after necrosis of the optic tract.

Thirty one patients had radiological check-ups 3 to 24 months (mean 11 months) after RS using angiography, MRI or CT scan (when check-up was done before the 12th month of follow up). Fifteen patients had more than one year of radiological follow-up. Ten patients have complete obliteration (3 between 9 and 13 months after RS); seven achieved a major obliteration (80% or more) of the AVM and six have a reduction of 50 to 80% of the lesion. According to the Spetzler grade, a major or total obliteration is obtained for 62% of the grade I–II AVMs (5/8 patients), 54% of the grade III (7/13) and 50% of the grade IV–V (5/10). Figure 2 illustrates the obliteration rate according to the time of check-up after RS. It confirms that some delay is required to obtain an obliteration. But some lesions can respond quickly to RS and 50% of the patients (8/16) have a reduction of 80% or more of their AVM 6 to 12 months after RS. Among the 15 patients who had more than 12 months of follow up, 80% (12/15) achieved a major or a complete obliteration.

Meningiomas

The mean clinical follow up after RS was 18 months (8 to 28 months). Thirteen patients are still alive without clinical evidence of disease with 4/9 presenting an improvement of tumour related symptoms. Two patients died, one from tumour re-growth and the other from progression of a breast sarcoma. Two grade 3 complications occurred 6 and 11 months after treatment: one hemiparesis plus right facial palsy and 1 severe visual impairment. Those 2 patients were treated for large lesions with 30 mm collimators. They both received 20 Gy. One of these received 50.4 Gy with EBRT before RS. Fourteen tumours had a CT check-up 4 to 24 months after treatment (RS or beginning of EBRT). Three tumours progressed 3, 9 and 11 months after treatment. One had RS for a third relapse with a very aggressive pathological lesion (multiple mitosis and very poorly differentiated cells) and died from continued progression. One of the 2 other progressions rapidly compressed the chiasma, the other one progressed outside the RS field (large multiple tumour);

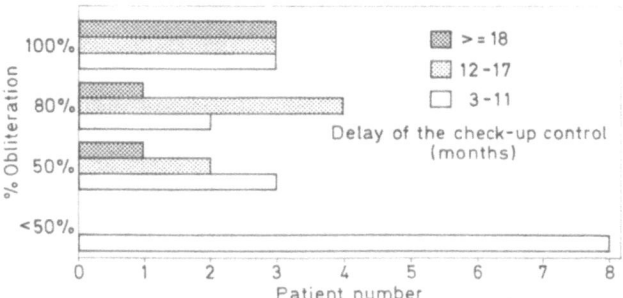

Fig. 2. Obliteration rate for 31 AVMs controlled 3 to 24 months after RS (angio, CT, or MRI)

both of them were cured by surgery. Five tumours seemed stabilised (with or without CT density modification) 4 to 22 months after treatment (4 with 12 to 22 months of follow up) and 6 others showed radiological regression. Figure 3 shows how this regression could be related to the initial size. The observed regressions seemed quicker after EBRT plus RS than after RS alone (mean of 6.5 versus 13.5 months).

Adenomas

The mean clinical follow up for the 36 adenomas was 21 months (9 to 31 months). Thirty one had a complete endocrine, radiological and visual evaluation 12 to 18 months after RS. Results are summarised in Table 5. Twelve patients developed visual complications with 4 grade 2 and 8 grade 3 complications. The grade 3 were 2 with bilateral blindness and 6 unilateral progressive blindness with a chiasmatic syndrome. The grade 2 complications were 2 chiasmatic syndromes with macula sparing and 2 minimal visual field and/or visual acuity reduction. For 7 of the 8 grade 3 compli-

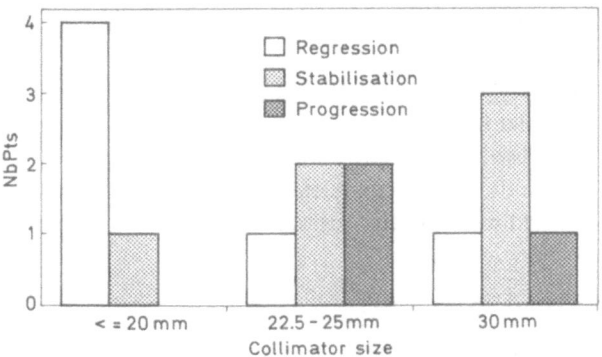

Fig. 3. 15 Mengiomas: response related to the SRT colimator size

Table 5. *Results of the RS for 31 Pituitary Adenomas Controlled 12 to 18 Months After Treatment*

Complication	−8 grade 3: 2 bilateral blindness + 6 unilateral blindness. (7/8 touching the chiasma) −4 grade 2: 2 chiasmatic syndrome + 2→ visual acuity/visual field. (2/4 touching the chiasma −19 without complication (3 touching the chiasma and 16 ⩾ 5 mm)
Radiologicaly	−9 size regressions −4 density changes −12 stable adenomas −6?
Biologicaly	−6 GH adenomas: 3 improved, 1 stable, 1 cured (pregnancy) −4 corticotropic adenomas: 2 cured, 2 improved at 1 year −16 patients with partial or without pituitary deficit before RS: 9 without deficit, 4 panhypopituitarism, 1 GH deficit, 1 TRH-GH deficit, 1 ACTH deficit (cure of the Cushing syndrome)

cations, the tumour was touching the chiasma and 4 showed radiation necrosis on MRI. Only 2 of the 4 grade 2 complications had a tumour in contact with the chiasma but the 2 others were large tumours. Only 3 of these 12 patients had normal visual field and normal vision before RS (1 grade 3 and 2 grade 2) and all 3 had large tumours. Ten of the 12 patients were treated with a large collimator of 22.5 to 30 mm. For the 19 patients without visual complications, only 3 had an adenoma touching the chiasma and for the sixteen others the chiasma was more than 5 mm distant from the adenoma. Radiologicaly, 9 adenomas regressed in size, a tumour density modification was observed in 4 and 12 were stable. For the 6 others, the imaging was not informative. Biologically, 5 of the 6 GH adenomas were stabilised or improved with one patient who became pregnant. All of the 4 controlled corticotropic adenomas were improved and probably cured after a longer follow up. Among the 16 patients with partial or without pituitary deficit, only 4 suffered complete hypopituitarism and 3 a partial hormonal deficit (with a cure for one case of Cushing's syndrome).

We did not evaluate the other cerebral lesions we treated by RS as the series are too small.

Discussion

All these results are, very preliminary as the mean follow up is only 14 to 21 months. The first point we can mention is the absence of new haemorrhage after 6 months post RS. The natural history of large AVMs would suppose a haemorrhage rate of approximately 3% per year [18] and we probably decreased this risk in our series. For AVMs, it would be useful to study the obliteration rate 2 or 3 years after RS. With all techniques, the total obliteration rate is from 70 to 85% at 2 years [10, 14, 18, 21, 22]. Our 80% (12/15) rate of obliteration of more than 80% of the AVM after 12 months (7/15 complete obliteration) and the obliteration of at least 50% of the volume of all the lesions lets us hope that we will achieve the same results even with initially large lesions which had, in the great majority, to be reduced by one or more courses of embolisation before they could be treated by RS. These embolisations do not seem to induce many more complications even if the complication rate of 7% (3/42) is in the higher range of the series reviewed by Larson *et al.* [11]. Although we did not deliver higher doses than 20 Gy at the periphery of the AVMs, we decided, since April 1992, to reduce the dose for lesions larger than 2 cm according to the Kjellberg monogram [6] and the Flickinger model [4] as all studies agree that the treated volume plays the major role in the incidence of complications after RS [4, 6, 17].

Few teams have a large experience in the treatment of meningiomas [1, 3, 9, 12]. A mean follow-up of 18 months is too short for these slowly growing tumours to arrive at conclusions on the role of RS in the control of the meningiomas of our series but the 4/9 clinical improvements associated with the 6/15 CT regressions and the 5 stabilisations (4 with more than 11 months of follow up) are very encouraging. These results are similar to the one year results of the Pittsburgh series [9]. The two complications due to radio-necrosis seem to confirm the high risk of RS previously noted for tumours [3, 17] and point out the necessity to reduce the doses or to fractionate the radiosurgical treatments. The association of EBRT to RS seems, in our series, to accelerate the regression and perhaps also the tumour control. A multicentric randomised trial would probably be interesting to compare fractionated radiosurgery to the association of conventional EBRT plus a single RS in the management of meningiomas unless other techniques like conformal radiotherapy show their benefits.

The treatment of pituitary adenomas was initiated on the basis of the Boston and Berkeley particles and the Swedish gamma-knife experiences [7, 8, 12, 13, 23, 24]. Our preliminary biological results are not disappointing with more than 50% of biological improvement for the secreting adenomas and 80% (25/31) of radiological stabilisations or regressions 12 to 18 months after RS. These results are absolutely comparable to the published series but not the complication rate we observed in our series which is much higher than the 2 to 4% previously described [7, 8, 12, 13] except for the induced hypopituitarism which was seen in about one third of the patients. In the face of these severe complications, we decided to stop RS for pituitary adenomas, which can be treated by EBRT, unless we could analyse and avoid the causes. The review of imaging and visual check-ups led to the conclusion that major visual complications occurred mostly when the tumour was close to the chiasma, larger than 2 cm and pre-therapeutic visual alterations were present. The published experience on pituitary RS do not define clearly the mean tumour volumes treated but it looks smaller and farther from the optic pathways. Even the central doses delivered were much higher, the tumour peripheral doses seemed lower than our 20 Gy. In the Berkeley experience [12], the treatment was also fractionated. Ganz also confirmed that non-secreting adenomas, usually larger than functional ones, are often too large to be treated by RS since patients generally present with visual symptoms [5] and signs.

Conclusion

This paper summarises the preliminary results of our RS experience with AVMs, meningiomas and pituitary adenomas. These results are very encouraging for AVMs and meningiomas. Deruty, one neurosurgeon specialising in AVM surgery, recently admitted that RS dramatically reduces the surgery rate and improves the neurological outcome for patients which used to be favourable (no or minor deficit) for 67% of patients before RS versus 90% with RS [2]. The reduction of the dose to between 20 and 15 Gy for lesions greater than 2 cm seems to decrease the risk of radionecroses, particularly for AVMs for which treatment will not be fractionated. The best treatment combination or fractionation has to be defined for meningiomas and other cerebral tumours but RS appears helpful in the management of non-surgical lesions. The complications observed for pituitary adenomas constrained us to stop RS treatments although clinical, biological and radiological results were good.

We are now developing a new technique that will allow fractionated treatment for tumours with an

acceptable reproducibility in order to deliver higher doses without increasing the complication rate and, in this way, to improve the local control, particularly for malignant tumours.

References

1. Coffey RJ, Lunsford LD (1990) Stereotactic radiosurgery using the 201 Cobalt-60 source gamma knife. Neurosurg Clin N Am 1: 933–953
2. Deruty R, Pelissou-Guyotat I, Mottolese C, Bascoulergue Y (1993) La place du neurochirurgien dans le traitement des malformations artério-veineuses cérébrales. Etude d'une série de 100 cas et revue de la littérature. Neurochirurgie 39: 212–224
3. Engenhart R, Kimmig BN, Hover KH, Wowra B, Sturm V, Van Kaick G, Wannenmacher M (1990) Stereotactic single high dose radiation therapy of benign intracranial meningiomas. Int J Radiat Oncol Biol Phys 19: 1021–1026
4. Flickinger JC (1989) An integrated logistic formula for prediction of complications from radiosurgery. Int J Radiat Oncol Biol Phys 17: 879–885
5. Ganz JC (1993) Gamma-knife applications in and around the pituitary fossa. In: Ganz JC (ed) Gamma-knife surgery. A guide for referring physicians. Springer, Wien New York, pp 122–132
6. Kjellberg RN (1979) Isoeffective dose parameters for brain necrosis in relation to proton radiosurgical dosimetry. In: Szikla G (ed) Stereotactic cerebral irradiation: INSERM Symposium no 12. Elsevier North Holland Amsterdam, pp 157–166
7. Kjellberg RN, Kliman B, Swisher B, Butler W (1984) Proton beam therapy of Cushing's disease and Nelson's syndrome. In: Black P McL (ed) Secretory tumours of the pituitary gland. Raven New York, pp 295–307
8. Kliman B, Kjellberg RN, Swisher B, Butler W (1994) Proton beam therapy of acromegaly: a 20-year experience. In: Black P McL (ed) Secretory tumours of the pituitary gland. Raven, New York, pp 191–211
9. Kondziolka D, Lunsford LD, Coffey RJ, Flickinger JC (1991) Stereotactic radiosurgery of meningiomas. J Neurosurg 74: 552–559
10. Larson DA, Gutin PH, Leibel SA, Philips TL, Sneed PK, Wara WM (1990) Stereotaxic irradiation of brain tumours. Cancer 65: 792–799
11. Larson DA, Wasserman TH, Drzymala RE, Simpson JR (1992) Stereotactic external beam irradiation. In: Perez CA, Brady LW (eds) Principles and practice of radiation oncology. Lippincott, Philadelphia, pp 553–563
12. Levy RP, Fabrikant JI, Frankel KA: Charged particle radiosurgery of the brain. Neurosurg Clin N Am 1: 955–990
13. Levy RP, Fabrikant JI, Frankel KA, Phillips MH, Lyma JT, Lawrence JH, Tobias CA (1990) Heavy-charged-particle radiosurgery of the pituitary gland: Clinical results of 840 patients. In: Proceedings of the European particle accelerator conference Nice, France
14. Loeffler JS, Alexander III E, Siddon RL, Saunders WM, Coleman CN, Winston KR (1989) Stereotactic radiosurgery for intracranial arteriovenous malformations using a standart linear accelerator. Int J Radiat Oncol Biol Phys 17: 673–677
15. Lutz W, Winston KR, Maleki N (1988) A system for stereotactic radiosurgery with a linear accelerator. Int J Radiat Oncol Biol Phys 14: 373–381
16. Muron T, Rocher FP, Sentenac I, Marquis I, Romestaing P, Gatignon D, Croisille M, Gerard JP (1993) La radiothérapie

stéréotaxique multifaisceaux. Expérience préliminaire d'une équipe lyonnaise. Ann Med Interne 144: 9–14

17. Nedzi L, Kooy H, Alexander III E, Gelman RS, Loeffler JS (1991) Variables associated with the development of complication from radiosurgery of intracranial tumors. Int J Radiat Oncol Biol Phys 21: 591–599

18. Ogilvy CS (1990) Radiation therapy for arteriovenous malformations: a review. Neurosurgery 26: 725–735

19. Saunders WM, Winston KR, Siddon RL, Svensson GH, Kijewski PK (1988) Radiosurgery for arteriovenous malformations of the brain using a standart linear accelerator: rationale and technique. Int J Radiat Oncol Biol Phys 15: 441–447

20. Sentenac I, Gerard JP, Martin P, Goutte R (1989) Radiothérapie des lésions intra-craniennes en conditions stéréotaxiques. XVIII congrès de la Société Française des Physiciens d'Hopitaux Lyon

21. Steinberg GK, Fabrikant JI, Marks MP, Levy RP, Frankel KA, Phillips MH, Shuer LM, Silverberg GD (1990) Stereotactic heavy-charged-particle Bragg-peak radiation for intracranial arteriovenous malformations. N Engl J Med 323: 96–101

22. Steiner L (1986) Radiosurgery in cerebral arteriovenous malformations. In: Flamm E Fein J (eds) Textbook of cerebrovascular surgery. Springer, New York, pp 1161–1215

23. Thoren M, Rähn T, Guo WY, Werner S (1991) Stereotactic radiosurgery with cobalt-60 gamma unit in the treatment of growth hormone producing pituitary tumors. Neurosurgery 29: 663–668

24. Thoren M, Sääf M, Degerblad M, Rähn T, Noren G, Bergstrand CG, Tallstedt L, Backlund EO (1988) Stereotactic irradiation for pituitary disease. Horm Res 30: 101–104

Correspondence: F. P. Rocher, Service de Radiotherapy, Centre Hospitalier Lyon-Sud, F-69310 Pierre Bénite, France.

Acta Neurochir (1995) [Suppl] 63: 115–118

Suction Fixation System for Stereotactic Radiosurgery of Intraocular Malignancies

M. Zehetmayer[1], R. Menapace[1], K. Kitz[2], and A. Ertl[2]

[1] Department of Ophthalmology, Oncology Service, and [2] Department of Neurosurgery, Gamma Knife Unit, University of Vienna, Wien, Austria

Summary

We designed a suction fixation system for the radiosurgical treatment of intraocular malignances with the Leksell gamma unit (gamma knife). Our device consists of a circular suction chamber and an adjustable unit to be fixed to the Leksell stereotactic head frame. All components are made of plastic materials in order to avoid artifacts in CT or MRT imaging. A permanent suction of 600 to 800 millibars is provided by a standard vacuum pump, powered by a portable battery. Suction times up to 40 minutes were well tolerated in all cases.

In the gamma knife of the Neurosurgical Department at the University of Vienna, we successfully used this device. Up to January 1994 we have performed 19 radiosurgical treatments in 9 patients with large or extra-large uveal melanomas and in one patient suffering from a choroidal metastasis.

Keywords: Suction fixation system; intraocular malignancies; uveal melanoma; radiosurgery.

Introduction

Radiotherapy of intraocular tumours includes brachytherapy with episcleral plaques (^{60}Co, ^{106}Ru, ^{125}I), megavoltage treatment and external beam irradiation with accelerated charged particles (helium ions, protons) [15]. Thermoradiotherapy is under experimental investigation [13].

Radiosurgery is well-established in the treatment of certain intracranial vascular lesions and small benign and malignant neoplasms [2,8,10,11,16]. With the Leksell stereotactic gamma unit (gamma knife, Model B, Elekta Instruments, Linköping, Sweden), the target is irradiated by focusing 201 highly collimated ^{60}Co sources, arranged in a hemispherical array [18].

In a rabbit eye melanoma model, irradiation with the gamma knife was capable of destroying the tumour-

provided the tumour was properly brought within focus and irradiated with 60 to 90 Gy [12]. In first experiences comprising 11 patients with uveal melanoma, a single-dose irradiation with the gamma knife seemed to be a promising treatment alternative to accelerated particle therapy [1]. Three retinoblastoma patients have been treated with the gamma knife and a total dose of 10 Gy was delivered within two sessions [17].

Absolute immobilisation of the target is an indispensible prerequisite for all stereotactic procedures. For treating uveal melanomas with the gamma knife, additional traction sutures with 5-0 silk through the four rectus muscles have been used [1].

We designed a noninvasive fixation method, using a suction attachment for safe and precise positioning of the eye during the radiosurgical procedure with the gamma knife.

Materials and Methods

The suction fixation system consists of a circular vacuum chamber and an adjustable unit to be fixed to the Leksell stereotactic head frame (Fig. 1). The vacuum chamber is similar to ophthalmic instruments used for stabilising the globe during keratoplasty and keratorefractive procedures [7,9]. The chamber's outer diameter is 24 mm, the aperture 12 mm. On the chamber's corneal side there is a ring-shaped vacuum area with an inner radius of 7.5 mm and an outer one of 9.5 mm (Fig. 2). This suction zone has 16 perforations, leading to a ring-shaped cavity which is connected to the suction pump by a silicone tube. The vacuum chamber is designed so as not to elevate intraocular pressure.

All components of the device are made of plastic materials which are permeable to radiation (polymethylmethacrylate for the vacuum chamber and polyamide for all other parts). This will avoid artifacts and thus optimize the delincation of the radiosurgical target during CT or MRT imaging (Fig. 3).

To keep suction time as short as possible, the Leksell stereotactic head frame is at first fixed to the skull. After retrobulbar anaesthesia with a 5 ccm solution of 2% lidocaine and 0.5% bupivacaine, stereotactic CT scanning is performed without the suction attachment. The primary co-ordinates, volume and extension of the malignancy are ascertained. The size of the collimator and, if necessary, a collimator plugging [4] is evaluated. The definitive stereotactic CT imaging with suction of the eye is performed only if the primary dose planning has been finished successfully. For this procedure, the vacuum chamber is inserted between the eye lids, placed centrally on the cornea and properly fixed to the limbus by a suction of 600 to 800 millibars. By means of two bolts, the chamber is connected to the adjustable fixation unit which is subsequently linked to the stereotactic head frame. The central aperture is filled with a lubricant to moisten the cornea (Fig. 4).

Any dislocation of the intraocular target during transportation and irradiation is prevented by a permanent suction of 600 to 800 millibars in the vacuum chamber. The vacuum pump is powered by a portable battery to allow patient's transport between the neuroradiological department and the gamma knife.

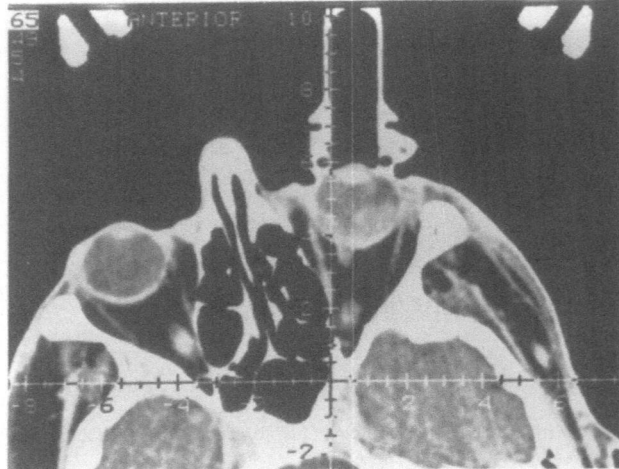

Fig. 3. Axial CT: a melanoma at the posterior pole, with the eye immobilized by the suction fixation system

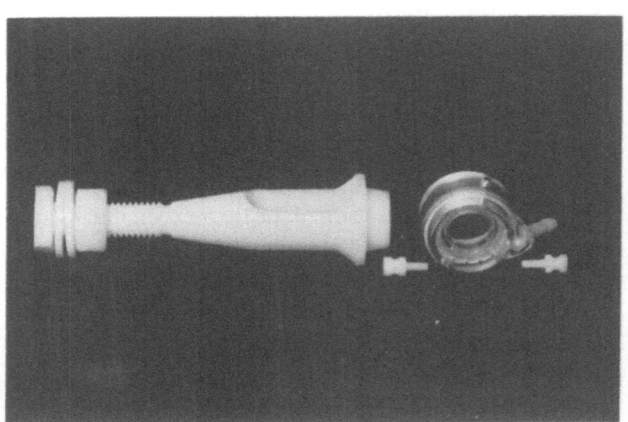

Fig. 1. Suction fixation system in a dismounted state

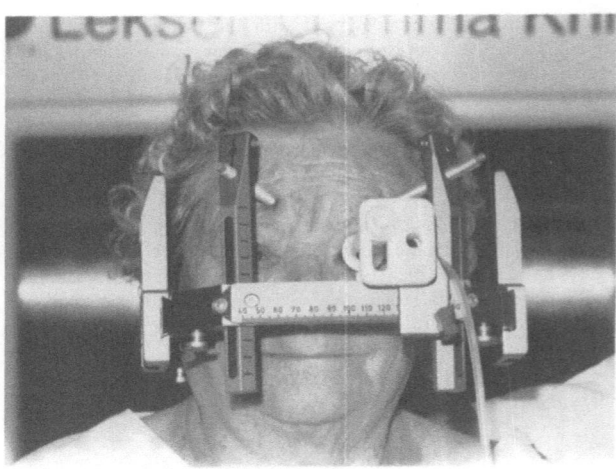

Fig. 4. Facial view: a patient prior to treatment

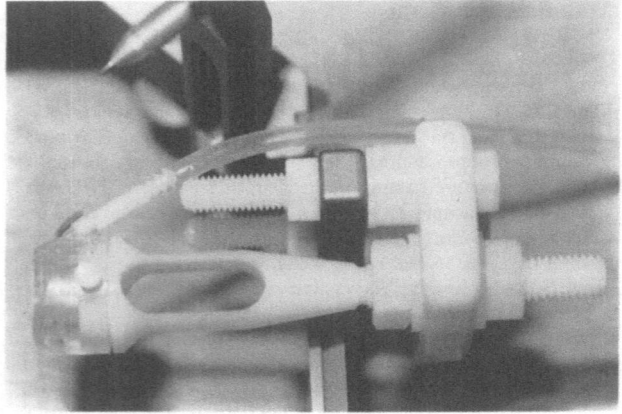

Fig. 2. Suction fixation system linked to the Leksell stereotactic head frame

Results

Until January 1994, we successfully performed 19 irradiation sessions. 9 patients with large or extra-large choroidal or ciliary body melanoma were irradiated with an average dose of 78 Gy ($+/-$ 18 Gy; range: 60 to 102 Gy) at the 50% isodose. In these patients the total dose was delivered in two procedures, mostly within 8 days.

In one additional case, an 83-year old woman suffering from multiple slowly growing metastases of an unknown primary tumour, a choroidal metastasis was irradiated in a single session with two shots and a dose of 25 Gy at the tumour border.

Suction times of no more than 40 minutes were well tolerated by all patients. In one case a lateral canthotomy had to be performed to allow the suction chamber to be inserted.

Using our technique, we were able to do radiosurgery for ocular lesions with the gamma knife, achieving the same high accuracy as in intracranial targets.

Immediately after the removal of the suction chamber moderate petechial subconjunctival haemorrhages corresponding to the shape of the vacuum area were noticed in all cases. They resolved within the first two days, without leaving any traces. In two cases small corneal erosions were observed when examined by slit lamp on the first postoperative day. However, they healed within two days.

Discussion

Ocular suction fixation techniques, such as suction contact lenses have been successfully used for the megavoltage treatment of retinoblastoma [14] or for the proton beam therapy of selected uveal melanomas [3,6]. Performing radiosurgery for intraocular malignancies, suction fixation techniques have considerable advantages compared to a surgical fixation of the globe by traction sutures through the rectus muscles [1].

Suction fixation systems are non-invasive. A gamma knife treatment with the suction fixation system is usually performed without any surgical procedures. No surgery-related complications will therefore occur.

A displacement of the globe into the orbit caused by resorption of the anaesthetic will not take place. The globe is safely immobilized and eye movements are completely excluded during delineation, dose planning and irradiation.

The very eccentric position of the eye within the Leksell head frame is a well-known problem which may prevent proper focusing of the intraocular malignancy within the gamma knife [5]. In comparison to the suture technique, a more posterior and therefore more favourable position of the intraocular target may be obtained by gently pressing the globe into the orbit.

The combination of our fixation technique with an adequate positioning of the head frame allows radiosurgical treatment of intraocular malignancies, in particular of the ciliary body-even in individuals with larger skulls.

Acknowledgement

This study was supported by an unrestricted grant from "Kampf der Blindheit", Vienna, Austria.

We are indebted to Mr. Rosner from Laserplast, Inc., Vienna, for producing the device and for such excellent cooperation.

References

1. Chinela AB, Zambrano A, Bunge HJ, Guevara JA, Antico JC, Alva O, Artes C, Coscia G (1992) Gamma knife radiosurgery in uveal melanomas. In: Steiner L (ed) Radiosurgery: baseline and trends. Raven, New York, pp 161–169
2. Coffey RJ, Lunsford LD, Flickinger JC (1992) The role of radiosurgery in the treatment of malignant brain tumors. Neurosurg Clin North Am 3: 231–244
3. Egger E, Zografos L, Perret C, Gailloud C (1993) Proton beam irradiation of choroidal melanomas at the PSI: technique and results. In: Alberti WE, Sagerman H (eds) Radiotherapy of intraocular and orbital tumors. Springer, Berlin Heidelberg New York Tokio, pp 57–72
4. Flickinger JC, Maitz A, Kalend A, Lundsford LD, Wu A (1990) Treatment volume shaping with selected beam blocking using the Leksell gamma unit. Int J Radiat Oncol Biol Phys 19: 783–789
5. Ganz JC (1993) Gamma knife surgery. Springer, Wien New York, 90: 147–148
6. Gragoudas ES, Goitein M, Koehler AM, Verhey L, Tepper J, Suit HD, Brockhurst R, Constable IJ (1977) Proton irradiation of small choroidal malignant melanomas. Am J Ophthal 83: 665–673
7. Hessburg P, Barron M (1980) A disposable trephine. Ophthalmic Surg 11: 730–733
8. Kondziolka D, Lunsford LD (1993) Radiosurgery of meningeomas. Neurosurg Clin North Am 3: 219–230
9. Krumeich JH, Grasl MM, Binder PS, Knülle A (1990) Geführtes Trepansystem für perforierende Keratoplastiken. In: Freyler H, Skorpik C, Grasl M (eds) 3. Kongress der Deutschen Gesellschaft für Intraokularlinsen-Implantation. Springer, Wien New York, pp 450–456
10. Linskey ME, Lunsford DL, Flickinger JC, Kondziolka D (1992) Stereotactic radiosurgery for acoustic tumours. Neurosurg Clin North Am 3: 191–205
11. Luxton G, Zbigniew P, Gabor J, Lucien A, Apuzzo LJM (1993) Stereotactic neurosurgery: principles and comparison of treatment methods. Neurosurgery 32: 214–259
12. Rand RW, Khonsary A, Brown WJ, Winter J, Snow HD (1987) Leksell stereotactic radiosurgery in the treatment of eye melanoma. Neurol Res 9: 142–146
13. Schipper J, Lagendijk JJW, Tan KEWP (1993) Hyperthermia in the treatment of intraocular tumours, in particular retinoblastoma. In: Alberti WE, Sagerman H (eds) Radiotherapy of intraocular and orbital tumors. Springer, Berlin Heidelberg New York Tokio, pp 57–72
14. Schipper J, Tan KEWP (1983) Management of retinoblastoma by precision megavoltage irradiation. In: Lommatzsch PK, Blodi FC (eds) Intraocular tumors. Springer, Berlin Heidelberg New York Tokio, pp 534–540
15. Shields JA, Shields CL (1992) Intraocular tumors: a text and atlas. Saunders, Philadelphia, pp 28–39
16. Steiner L, Linquist C, Adler JR, Torner JC, Steiner M (1992) Clinical outcome of radiosurgery for cerebral arteriovenous malformations. J Neurosurg 77: 1–8

17. Trampe EB, Backlund EO, Bergström M, Greitz T, Kock E, Lax I, Lundell G, Tengroth B (1983) Results obtained in treating retinoblastoma patients with different techniques at the Karolinska Hospital. In: Lommatzsch PK, Blodi FC (eds) Intraocular tumors. Springer, Berlin Heidelberg New York Tokio, pp 529–533

18. Wu A (1992) Physics and dosimetry of the gamma knife. Neurosurg Clin North Am 3: 35–50

Correspondence: Martin Zehetmayer, M.D., Department of Ophthalmology, Oncology Service, Spitalgasse 2, A-1090 Wien, Austria.

Index of Keywords

C. Lindquist, D. Kondziolka, J. S. Loeffler (eds.)

Advances in Radiosurgery

Proceedings of the 1st Congress of the International Stereotactic Radiosurgery Society, Stockholm 1993

1994. 71 figures. VIII, 124 pages.
Cloth DM 150,–, öS 1050,–
Reduced price for subscribers to "Acta Neurochirurgica":
Cloth DM 135,–, öS 945,–
ISBN 3-211-82612-2

(Acta Neurochirurgica, Supplement 62)

Radiosurgery is a rapidly developing form of minimally invasive neurosurgery. Selected papers from the first meeting of the International Stereotactic Radiosurgery Society in Stockholm, June 1993, reflect current multidisciplinary approaches to difficult intracranial neurosurgical problems. Neurosurgeons, radiotherapists, oncologists, radiobiologists, physicists and representatives of several other clinical disciplines inform about the state-of-the-art of radiosurgical treatment of a multitude of intracranial problems such as arteriovenous malformations, pituitary and pineal tumors, vestibular schwannomas as well as metastatic brain tumors and gliomas.

Prices are subject to change without notice

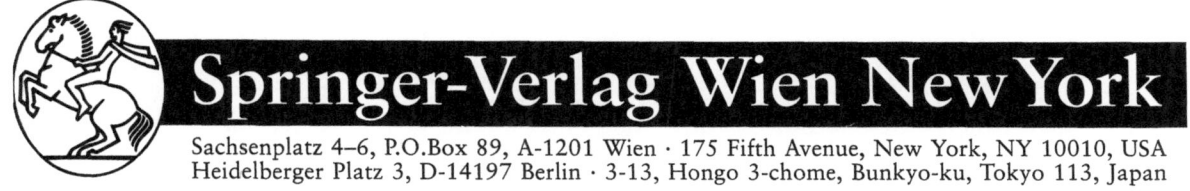

Springer-Verlag Wien New York

Sachsenplatz 4–6, P.O.Box 89, A-1201 Wien · 175 Fifth Avenue, New York, NY 10010, USA
Heidelberger Platz 3, D-14197 Berlin · 3-13, Hongo 3-chome, Bunkyo-ku, Tokyo 113, Japan

C. Lindquist, D.E. Leksell, K.S. Rocklage (eds)

Advances in Radiosurgery

Proceedings of the 1st Congress of the International
Stereotactic Radiosurgery Society, Stockholm 1993

Springer-Verlag
and the Environment

WE AT SPRINGER-VERLAG FIRMLY BELIEVE THAT AN international science publisher has a special obligation to the environment, and our corporate policies consistently reflect this conviction.

WE ALSO EXPECT OUR BUSINESS PARTNERS – PRINTERS, paper mills, packaging manufacturers, etc. – to commit themselves to using environmentally friendly materials and production processes.

THE PAPER IN THIS BOOK IS MADE FROM NO-CHLORINE pulp and is acid free, in conformance with international standards for paper permanency.